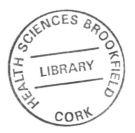

Education for Patients and Clients

Patient education is fundamental to good health care practice, but often undervalued as a nursing intervention. In *Education for Patients and Clients* Vivien E. Coates explains how education contributes to holistic nursing practice, directly improving health care outcomes and enabling patients to become more active participants in their own care.

Pulling together research from both education and health care, the book sets out the theoretical background to educating patients and investigates strategies for making interventions as effective as possible. Subjects covered include:

- learning theories
- teaching strategies
- patients with long-term health problems
- promoting behavioural change

Education for Patients and Clients provides a much needed resource for nurses wishing to develop their practice in this area and will be essential reading for all courses relating to education in health care.

Vivien E. Coates is Senior Lecturer in Nursing at the University of Ulster.

Routledge Essentials for Nurses cover four key areas of nursing:

- core theoretical studies
- psychological and physical care
- nurse education
- new directions in nursing and health care

Written by experienced practitioners and teachers, books in this series encourage a critical approach to nursing concepts and show how research findings are relevant to nursing practice.

The series editors are **Robert Newell**, University of Leeds and **David Thompson**, University of York and Nursing Advisor at the Department of Health.

Also in this series:

Education for Patients and Clients

Vivien E. Coates

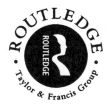

London and New York

i16718294

First published 1999
by Routledge
2 Park Square, Milton Park, Abingdon, Oxon, OX14 4RN
Simultaneously published in the USA and Canada
by Routledge
270 Madison Ave, New York NY 10016

Routledge is an imprint of the Taylor & Francis Group

Transferred to Digital Printing 2006

Typeset in Times New Roman by
The Florence Group

British Library Cataloguing in Publication Data
A catalogue record for this book is available from the British Library

Library of Congress Cataloging in Publication Data
Coates, Vivien E. (Vivien Elizabeth), 1957–
   Education for patients and clients / Vivien E. Coates.
   p. cm. – (Routledge essentials for nurses)
   Includes bibliographical references and index.
   1. Patient education. I. Title. II. Series.
   [DNLM: 1. Patient Education–methods Nurses' Instruction.
   W 85 C652e 1999]
   RT90.C63 1999
   615.5'071–dc21
   DNLM/DLC for Library of Congress 99–17634
                                        CIP

ISBN 0–415–14849–9 (hbk)
ISBN 0–415–14850–2 (pbk)

Contents

Illustrations

Figures

Table

Chapter 1

Education for patients and clients

What this book is about

Patient education is exciting and creative but has yet to reach its full potential as an integrated part of nursing practice. For many reasons it is vital that nurses develop this aspect of their work to make it a unique and identifiable part of nursing. In spite of the need to exploit the potential of patient education it is an activity which can often be overshadowed by other items on nursing's busy agenda. There are so many demands on nurses' time that, even with the best will in the world, patient education may not receive the careful attention which it deserves.

This book has been written with the aim of nurturing interest and enthusiasm for patient education. This can be a fascinating subject but, like so many other aspects of nursing practice, may be regarded as something which we get on with when we have time, often without examining the underlying scientific foundation for practice. Patient education may at first glance appear to be a simple activity, but in reality it can be a difficult, exacting and enormously challenging aspect of care.

This book is meant to act as a prompt to raise the priority given to patient education at a practical level and has been written to serve several purposes. First, it draws together a wide range of material on patient education and can be used as a literature review for nurses who are too busy to undertake such a search themselves. Second, this book outlines a range of educational approaches and can help nurses to appreciate that although there is no consensus on how sick people learn or how we can best promote behavioural change, we must not ignore learning theories, which may be able to guide practice. For people in an appropriate position to do so there is an urgent need for theory to be used and tested in practice with the aim of further developing the theoretical basis for patient education. Third, this book presents evidence, where possible, which can be used to underpin nursing activity and can therefore make a contribution towards evidence-based practice. When the body of literature on patient education is consulted there is a paradoxical situation in which, on the one hand, there is a great deal written on patient education, yet on the other hand, there is still a lot we do not know about how individuals with a health problem learn and about the most effective and valuable teaching interventions which we should be offering. In this book points for good practice which can be supported by evidence are presented. As nurses we must be able to discuss and justify the rationale for our practice and also to demonstrate that it has a therapeutic effect upon clients.

Introduction to Chapter I

This chapter sets the scene for the rest of the book. The notion of patient education as it relates to this book will be defined and clarified. The scope of the book will be outlined, and those areas which are included and those which are excluded will be mentioned. In a short work such as this one, it is not possible to cover all aspects of patient education at a level which would allow for meaningful debate, and so, of necessity, some areas are covered in greater depth than others. The need for patient education will be discussed and supported through reference to research. The role of patients participating in their own health care will be discussed and the case made that people cannot hope to be involved in decisions about their care without an adequate knowledge base. In this chapter, and indeed throughout the book, it is intended to encourage readers to examine their own views on patient education. We often set out with whole sets of assumptions which we have never really stopped to look at. It is hoped that this process of reflection will increase enthusiasm and knowledge about this important aspect of patient care.

The scope of this book

In this book it is intended to give a broad overview of general issues and principles of patient education which may be applied widely, rather than relate to any specific patient need or clinical condition. Second, the book will focus on the needs of adults rather than children. The needs of these two age groups are quite different and cannot be readily covered in one work. Third, the book will refer to patients whose primary diagnosis relates to physical disease rather than mental health problems, although many of the issues discussed will be common between these two groups. Fourth, the needs of patients/clients are the primary concern rather than those of their relatives. Once again, much of the material regarding education may well apply to relatives as well as patients, and the needs of relatives form an important subject. However, there is a quite different literature regarding this area of education, and this is beyond the remit of this book.

Indeed, it is acknowledged that all the groups which are 'excluded' from this book have very important educational needs. The reasons for not including them are the need to complete a book which is comparatively brief and the need to keep the content focused rather than trying to cover all aspects of patient education at a superficial level within a single volume. There is a vast amount of material relating to all these topics and to look at some issues in depth the scope of the book needed to be limited and defined. However, many of the points raised and the research cited will also be readily applicable to the needs of groups other than physically ill patients.

Defining patient education

In the current literature there appears to be overlap and confusion relating to the broader concepts of health promotion and health education in relation to patient education. For example, is health promotion the same as health education and how does patient education relate to these activities? Where does one activity end and the next one begin? There is by no means a consensus of opinion regarding definitions of these activities (Caraher, 1998, 1994). Latter *et al.* (1992) offer a helpful analysis in which health promotion is interpreted as relating to health policy at local and national levels to influence health in its broadest interpretation. In this sense it relates to primary prevention of disease and ill health and to promoting good health to the population at large. Although the World Health Organization (1987) states that health promotion should also be about 'the process of enabling people to increase control over and improve their health' they remind us that this should be thought of as occurring at individualised rather than political levels. Health education is visualised by Latter *et al.* (1992) as embracing patient education, information-giving, healthy lifestyle advice and encouraging patient and family participation in care. Thus patient education may be viewed as a part of health education.

In contrast, Caraher (1998: 56) suggests that health education

> is that which occurs when individuals are not patients. . . . The focus is on the promotion of health rather than the treatment of illness and the relationship is more than that of the health promotion scenario.

It would appear then, that health promotion, health education and patient education can be viewed as different activities, although patient education is itself a means of promoting health.

However, what is meant by the words *patient education* is also not immediately clear. There are many definitions of patient education available, since most articles and books on this subject include a definition to guide the reader in the interpretation of the material presented. When reviewing the definitions it can be seen that there are a wide variety of terms, phrases and meanings associated with this subject. Wilson-Barnett (1988) has carefully examined the differences amongst the commonly used terms: information-giving, teaching, education and counselling. These are not the same processes and can be expected to have different outcomes. She warns that careless or confused use of these terms may lead to inadequate understanding and practice. Falvo (1985: 3) also notes the variation in terms used:

> The terms *patient education* and *patient teaching* have been used synonymously. The term *instruction* has been used interchangeably with *education*. *Patient education* has in some instances been equated with *patient information*.

Rankin and Duffy Stallings (1990) distinguish between patient teaching and education. They indicate that patient teaching is the giving of information and thus has a narrower remit than patient education, which includes information-giving but also embraces interpreting and using the information and influencing attitudes and behaviour. This view would concur with an analysis of the concept presented by Falvo (1985).

The following definition, developed by Squyres (1980: 1) from the work of Green *et al.* (1980), will be used to orientate the reader to the focus of this book. Patient education is the

planned combinations of learning activities designed to assist
people who are having or have had experience with illness or disease in making changes in their behaviour conducive to health.

If we stop to analyse this statement we can learn several important
points:

1   the process of patient education is a **planned** rather than a
    random process
2   a **combination** rather than a single event or intervention is
    required
3   the purpose is to **assist** rather than to force or demand people
    to change behaviour
4   patient teaching is related to **disease or illness** in contrast to
    health promotion or health education which can also be aimed
    at healthy people
5   **behavioural change** conducive to health, not just an increase
    in knowledge, is often an overall goal

These points will be referred to throughout this book as major
themes which must be borne in mind when considering the topic
of patient education. Patient education has often been criticised as
being authoritative but this definition implies a helping rather than
a dominating role. To illustrate that this definition is still relevant
in today's health care climate a much more recent definition is also
given, which is in essence the same, although a bit more detailed
than the one given above.

> Patient education is planned, organized learning experiences
> designed to facilitate voluntary adoption of behaviours or beliefs
> conducive to health. It is a set of planned educational activi-
> ties that are separate from clinical patient care. The activities
> of a patient education program must be designed to attain goals
> the patient has participated in formulating. The primary focus
> of these activities includes acquisition of information, skills,
> beliefs and attitudes which impact on health status, quality of
> life, and possibly health care utilization.
>
> (Burckhardt, 1994: 2)

Once again, it will be noted that the ideas of planning, ongoing
activity, patient collaboration and behaviour change are clearly parts

of this definition. The notion that teaching is related to health and illness is implicit within it, although not explicitly stated.

It is hoped that these definitions clearly portray the vision of patient education which is the focus of this book. Finally, for the purposes of clarity, following the approach of Professor Wilson-Barnett (1988) the term *patient* is used to indicate that this book is focusing on the educational needs of people with a medically diagnosed condition.

The need for patient education

There are many good reasons why patient education is considered to be important and four particularly pertinent reasons will be explored in this chapter. They are:

- the nature of disease and illness prevalent in our society is changing
- patient participation is a fashionable concept in health care which can only be achieved if there is adequate patient education
- there is research evidence to suggest that patient education is an effective intervention in a wide variety of settings
- there is research evidence that patients want to receive education about their health problems

The changing nature of disease and illness in society

The pattern of disease in prosperous countries has changed during this century (Kiger, 1995). Environmental reforms, together with improvements in diet, revolutionised chances for the general public to remain healthy (Allen and Hall, 1988). Reforms regarding sanitation, water, housing and working conditions resulted in an increased life expectancy. This has, in turn, caused a shift towards disease affecting the elderly (Department of Health, 1995, 1997). The number of deaths from diseases which may have a strong social component and a multi-factorial aetiology, such as cancer and heart disease, have also increased. As a result of such changes in the nature of health and illness medical intervention is now called upon to treat conditions which are often not immediately life threatening. Rather they prevent individuals from leading fully independent lives. Rapid interventions such as surgery are often not appropriate;

instead, the treatment of chronic conditions may require the patient to undertake a prolonged regime of self-management (Fitzpatrick *et al.*, 1984).

Table 1.1 from *On the State of the Public Health* (D.o.H., 1995) illustrates the five main causes of death for males and females in England in 1994. The overall figures (column 1) illustrate that ischaemic heart disease, cerebro-vascular accident, malignant disease of the respiratory system, pneumonia, and malignant disease of the digestive organs and peritoneum were the five major categories of death. All these categories of disease would require major health care provision in the form of treatment and management. It would be fair to say that all these diseases would offer health care professionals ample opportunity for patient education from diagnosis until eventual death. Such education would span community and acute hospital services and outpatient settings and could involve a multitude of health care professionals.

In the last century infectious diseases were a major cause of mortality. The incidence of diseases such as scarlet fever, measles, whooping cough, diphtheria, typhoid, and tuberculosis was relatively high (Kiger, 1995). Until the 1980s, deaths from infectious diseases were thought to be declining; however, the acquired immuno-deficiency syndrome (AIDS) epidemic has demonstrated that infection may still be a major threat to health. In England in 1994 1,634 cases of AIDS were reported. Since 1982 a total of 9,510 cases of AIDS have been reported, of whom 6,434 are known to have died (D.o.H., 1995: 159). People with this condition will need appropriate health care intervention. Clearly, this will include patient education.

The strategy for *The Health of the Nation* (D.o.H., 1992a) was developed to try to target resources most appropriately to attempt to prevent ill-health, or if necessary, to treat it. The key target areas of the strategy are coronary heart disease and stroke, cancers, mental illness, HIV/AIDS and sexual health and reducing the mortality due to accidents. All these key areas will require patient education initiatives if there is to be any chance of the targets being met. Documents such as those mentioned above help to illustrate the nature of disease prevalent in our society, and presumably are similar to those of many other countries of the western world. On the basis of such statistics it can be argued that patient education must remain a priority area in the work of health care professionals.

In addition, recent health policy such as *The Health of the Nation* and *A Vision for the Future* (D.o.H., 1993) recommends the

Table 1.1 Five main causes of death for males and females at different ages (and percentages[1] of all causes of deaths), England, 1994

Rank	All ages – 1 and over		1–14 years		15–34 years		35–54 years		55–74 years		75 years and over	
	Males	Females	Males	Females	Males	Females	Males	Females	Males	Females	Males	Females
1	410–414 Ischaemic heart disease 28%	410–414 Ischaemic heart disease 22%	E800–E999 External causes of injury and poisoning 30%	E800–E999 External causes of injury and poisoning 25%	E950–E959 Suicide and undetermined injury† 24%	E950–E959 Suicide and undetermined injury† 12%	410–414 Ischaemic heart disease 24%	174 MN* of female breast 19%	410–414 Ischaemic heart disease 32%	410–414 Ischaemic heart disease 22%	410–414 Ischaemic heart disease 26%	410–414 Ischaemic heart disease 23%
2	430–438 Cerebro-vascular disease 8%	430–438 Cerebro-vascular disease 13%	140–239 Neoplasms 19%	140–239 Neoplasms 17%	E810–E819 Motor vehicle traffic accidents 17%	E810–E819 Motor vehicle traffic accidents 11%	150–159 MN* of digestive organs and peritoneum 9%	179–189 MN* of genito-urinary organs 9%	162 MN* of trachea, bronchus and lung 11%	150–159 MN* of digestive organs and peritoneum 9%	480–486 Pneumonia 11%	430–438 Cerebro-vascular disease 15%
3	162 MN* of trachea, bronchus and lung 8%	480–486 Pneumonia 11%	320–389 Diseases of the nervous system and sense organs 11%	740–759 Congenital anomalies 14%	E850–E869 Accidental poisoning by drugs, medica-ments and biologicals 6%	174 MN* of female breast 6%	E950–E959 Suicide and undeter-mined injury† 7%	150–159 MN* of digestive organs and peritoneum 8%	150–159 MN* of digestive organs and peritoneum 10%	430–438 Cerebro-vascular disease 8%	430–438 Cerebro-vascular disease 11%	480–486 Pneumonia 14%

Rank	All ages – 1 and over		1–14 years		15–34 years		35–54 years		55–74 years		75 years and over	
	Males	Females	Males	Females	Males	Females	Males	Females	Males	Females	Males	Females
4	150–159 MN* of digestive organs and peritoneum 8%	150–159 MN* of digestive organs and peritoneum 6%	460–519 Diseases of the respiratory system 10%	320–389 Diseases of the nervous system and sense organs 10%	001–139 Infectious and parasitic diseases 5%	200–208 MN* of lymphatic and haematopoietic tissue 5%	162 MN* of trachea, bronchus and lung 7%	410–414 Ischaemic heart disease 7%	430–438 Cerebrovascular disease 6%	162 MN* of trachea, bronchus and lung 8%	490–496 Chronic obstructive pulmonary disease and allied conditions 7%	415–429 Diseases of pulmonary circulation and other forms of heart disease 6%
5	480–486 Pneumonia 7%	415–429 Diseases of pulmonary circulation and other forms of heart disease 5%	740–759 Congenital anomalies 9%	460–519 Diseases of the respiratory system 9%	200–208 MN* of lymphatic and haematopoietic tissue 4%	179–189 MN* of genito-urinary organs 5%	430–438 Cerebrovascular disease 4%	162 MN* of trachea, bronchus and lung 6%	490–496 Chronic obstructive pulmonary disease and allied conditions 6%	174 MN* of female breast 7%	150–159 MN* of digestive organs and peritoneum 6%	150–159 MN* of digestive organs and peritoneum 5%
Remainder	41%	43%	22%	25%	46%	62%	48%	50%	35%	45%	39%	36%
All causes of death	247852	265917	941	692	5965	2467	17419	11505	100033	67962	123494	183291

Source: OPCS/ONS

Notes

1 May not add up to 100 due to rounding.   * MN = malignant neoplasm.

† Suicide and undetermined injury = (E950–E959) and (E980–E989), excluding E988.8

promotion of self-care in the National Health Service. This trend is reflected in the shift from hospital to community health care. Hospital services used to dominate health care but as health care needs increase and become more complex community based care has gained greater status. The recent report *The New NHS: Modern – Dependable* (D.o.H., 1997) indicates that this trend is set to continue and to be developed. According to Baggott (1994: 202) 'around 90 per cent of illness is managed outside hospital'. The shift in the provision of care will necessitate patients taking greater responsibility for their health and to do so they will require sufficient and appropriate education.

The rise of patient participation in health care

The context in which health care is provided, reflecting contemporary views about patients' roles and needs, gives rise to the second suggested reason why patient education is thought to be so important. The culture in which health care is provided helps shape the nature of the service. In the late 1990s concepts such as patient participation, empowerment, self-care, patients as partners in care, active rather than passive patients, are widely discussed and generally taken to be good ideas. It is no longer politically correct to assume that patients will 'do as they are told'.

The concept of patient participation is highly relevant to the subject of patient education as patients can only participate if they have the ability to do so. Thus education is a prerequisite to participation. In addition to this, education is more relevant if it is assumed that patients are to be actively involved in their health care. If patients are expected to do as they are told why spend time educating them about their condition? Although patient participation is a fashionable concept it remains a controversial topic in practice as opinions vary widely about the role that patients should adopt. At one extreme is the view in which supremacy of the professionals is supported, as is parodied by Brody in his depiction of the traditional passive patient's only obligation as being '*to seek competent help and co-operate with the physician in order to get well*' (Brody, 1980: 718). Whilst few may admit allegiance to such a perspective, strategies to limit patient choice can still be found in current health care practice (Draper, 1996). At the other extreme is the call for autonomous patients who are considered to be full partners with health care professionals. However, this is difficult to achieve in practice due to knowledge and power differentials prevalent in conventional health care settings (May, 1995) as will be discussed later in this chapter.

Clarifying the meaning of patient participation in care

Terms such as patient participation, self-help, self-care and consumer participation are frequently cited; they may relate to the same issue, or perhaps to rather different topics. Greenfield *et al.* (1985) noted a lack of agreement among researchers in the area of 'patient participation' in care. They suggest that patient participation requires more than compliance with the medical regimen, and has more to do with involvement in the health care professional–patient interaction. Brownlea (1987) suggested that participation should be taken to mean becoming actively involved in the decision-making process, or being consulted on an issue or matter. This view is supported by others, such as Steele *et al.* (1987) who believe that 'active' patients ask questions, seek explanations, state preferences, offer opinions and expect to be heard. These are all activities which contribute to the process of education. Moreover, it is likely that active participation itself requires considerable education of the patient.

Power and participation

If nurses and patients are to work as partners it implies that they should have equal power in the relationship, or at least that patients must have some power. Traditionally patients have been relatively powerless while health care professionals have been powerful. For example:

> The classical view of medicine places the patient in the passive role of recipient of drugs, advice and treatment with the doctor on his lofty pedestal dispensing 'the truth' and remedies (often of questionable value and rarely understood by the purveyors) with god-like omniscience.
>
> (Walford and Alberti, 1985: 200)

Although an extreme view it holds some truth and can also be said to apply to health professionals other than doctors. Hewison (1995) conducted a non-participant study of the way nurses may use language to exert power over patients. His results led him to conclude that nurses do exert power over their patients and use language as a means of doing so. His findings are supported by the research by Draper (1996). Power can be transferred to patients (Rodwell, 1996) and this technique, sometimes referred to as empowerment, is valuable in the repertoire of patient education skills and will be discussed in Chapter 7. More important, perhaps, are the beliefs and attitudes of nurses, as it is only if nurses believe that patients have a right to power that it is worth considering the means by which this can be achieved. Appropriate patient education may be one such means.

It can also be argued that there is a moral component to the issue of patient participation. For example, Ashworth *et al.* (1992: 1438) suggest that: 'To be insufficiently attentive to what have been shown to be the requirements of participation places the nurse or other health care professional in danger of treating the patient as less than a proper human being.' Porter (1994) has written about the importance of nurse–patient relationships which have attempted to give patients more power and make them more of an equal partner. This, Porter believes, 'accredits patients with the full humanity that is their due' (274).

To what extent do patients want to participate in health care?

While it may be argued that patients should participate actively in the maintenance of their health, it is important to know whether such individuals want to undertake this role. Thompson *et al.* (1993) investigated the extent to which 459 people wanted to be involved in making decisions about their own medical treatment. They found, as predicted, that individuals wanted to participate in care which did not require medical expertise but were wary of being involved in decision making that did. Clearly, people recognise that they cannot participate in care if they lack appropriate information or experience.

Similarly, Avis (1994) reports the results of a small but interesting study to gain insight into patients' perceptions of their participation in making decisions about a forthcoming minor surgical intervention. All twelve subjects preferred the doctor or nurse to decide upon the most appropriate course of action in recognition of their greater knowledge and experience of the subject area. From the data it appeared that the patients expected to be told what was going to be involved in their treatment rather than given choices about it. However, had the patients been more knowledgeable, it might have been possible for them to engage in the planning of their own health care to a greater degree.

Hack *et al.* (1994: 279) also investigated relationships between 'involvement in making treatment decisions and preferences for information about diagnosis, treatment, side effects and prognosis' in a study involving 35 women with breast cancer. They found that women who wanted an active decision-making role also wanted detailed information about their condition. However, passively oriented people demonstrated no clear relationship about desire for information. The authors concluded that research is required into active and passive roles of patients and the impact they have on disease progression and psychological well-being.

Anecdotal accounts from patients are also available. For example, Mara Flaherty (1981) describes her experiences over the previous fourteen years whilst suffering from cancer. She advocates those with cancer being encouraged to participate in their own care and in the decision-making process:

> it has taken me many years to change from passive patient to active participant. It took time, some dreadful experiences . . . and enrolment in a structured education programme before I began to be a full partner.
>
> (Flaherty, 1981: 25)

For her the most important reason for making this transition was that it gave her an element of control in her destiny. The power of control helped to reduce feelings of vulnerability, 'otherwise it appears that one's destiny is solely in the hands of health care providers' (ibid.). However, it should be remembered that while anecdotal reports may be valid, they do not bear the authority of findings generated through systematic research processes.

In contrast to the studies cited above, May (1995) challenges the view that patients wish to be active partners in care. He raises the important point that patients may not view themselves as active partners in their care, nor as experts on their health. Such people may resist these ideas, possibly at the risk of being labelled non-compliant. May warns us against assuming that the work of theorists can be transformed into practice. All such theories need to be tested.

Many attempts to elaborate upon and clarify patients' views on this issue have been made (Steele *et al.*, 1987; Waterworth and Luker, 1990; Rourke, 1991; Biley, 1992) but results are inconclusive. This may be due to weaknesses in the research designed to investigate these issues, such as focusing on different target populations, diverse methods of investigation used or confusing terminology. To help obtain a clearer picture it is important that terms such as *patient participation* are clarified, and that research designed to investigate these subjects is rigorous.

From the literature available it would appear that active participation in health care cannot be assumed to be the goal of all patients. When the outcome of the decision is very important and carries considerable responsibility or risk, individuals may be willing to let others be in charge, since such responsibility may be a burden (Steele *et al.*, 1987). However, people who are ignorant of the necessary information to make decisions are denied the opportunity to be active participants in care.

Additionally, the needs of chronically ill people, who are often obliged to bear responsibility for the daily management of a condition which affects their health and well-being should be considered. Participation in their own care is often a reality and a necessity for these people, rather than a choice (Peyrot *et al.*, 1987).

Perhaps the conclusion to be drawn from the available research is that allowance for individual preference must be made. Such a view would be endorsed by Slack (1977); Steele *et al.* (1987); Brearley (1990); and Waterworth and Luker (1990).

Framework for participation

The framework suggested by Szasz and Hollender (1956) may still serve as a useful guide in practice even though it is now rather dated. It embraces three models to explain the relationship between patient and physician, and as such indicates that the relationship is not static.

First they proposed an activity passivity model, which might often be considered the traditional approach to health care. In it the patient is the passive recipient of the treatment actively prescribed by the physician. In other words the doctor 'does something to' the patient such as surgery, anaesthesia, or prescribing medication. Szasz and

Hollender suggest that it is the most appropriate approach to use in acute and emergency situations when treatment is decided and undertaken without a contribution from the patient. The appropriateness of allocating a purely passive patient role in all acute illnesses can, of course, be challenged.

Second, the guidance co-operation model was proposed as a framework for non-emergency situations. Although the patients needed treatment for a particular problem, they were conscious and had feelings and goals which needed to be taken into account. Whilst the doctor knew more about the situation than the patient, both people would contribute to the relationship.

The third model proposed was that of mutual participation. In this type of interaction it would be important for both persons to have equal power, to need each other, and to engage in activity that would in some way satisfy both parties. This model would be favoured by those patients wanting to be active in their own care. This would appear to be a realistic approach when considering the treatment of chronic disease: patients' own experiences might provide reliable and important clues to therapy. As treatment was mainly carried out by the patient, the essential role of the health professional was to facilitate self-management practices among patients. The model of mutual participation embraces notions of friendship and the imparting of expert advice.

The appropriateness of each level of activity depends upon the type of health problem. It would appear that patient passivity is normal in acute illness, but is potentially dysfunctional in chronic illness (Szasz and Hollender, 1956). This framework offers a flexible and valuable way of considering the role of patients in health care, rather than adopting a single approach in which only one patient role is endorsed. More recently, Caraher (1994) and others have supported the typology they attribute to Roter (1987), which includes the following three approaches to patient education: authoritative guidance, active participation and independent decision making. This typology appears similar to the work of Szasz and Hollender but patients have a more active and dominant role throughout.

Patient education: an effective intervention

The third reason why patient education is advocated derives from research results which demonstrate that it can be an effective intervention. Due to the rising costs of health care greater emphasis is now placed on efficiency and effectiveness of services. According to Baggott (1994) an effective service 'is one which produces a desirable health outcome, for example, patients who recover from an operation' (48) while efficiency 'is achieved where output is maximised from a given input of resources' (49). Neither of these qualities is easy to demonstrate. However, if patient education is to be advocated it must be demonstrated that it is both an efficient and effective therapy for patients.

In financial terms Bartlett (1989) reports that patient education is worthwhile in that it can lower costs and improve quality of care. For example, 'when linked with discharge planning, patient education can facilitate earlier discharge' (88). More recently, he conducted a cost-benefit analysis involving twelve studies which met his specific criteria and concluded that 'on average, for every dollar invested in patient education, \$3–4 were saved' (89).

The work of Roach *et al.* (1995) also supports the view that patient education is an efficient intervention. They report the findings of a study in which pre-operative assessment and education was offered to 463 patients requiring joint replacement. Three hundred people attended the programme over a 21-month period. The authors report that after the programme the average length of stay in hospital was shortened by a day, which represents a decrease of 19.5 per cent in patient hospitalisation. When multiplied by the number of patients this was estimated to represent an annual saving in gross charges of \$763,866. It was thought that by being more knowledgeable and feeling less anxious patients were more in control of their care. The report concludes with the following:

> In this era of health reform, it is essential for nursing to find ways to cut costs, yet strive to provide excellent patient care. By providing education pre-operatively, we have not only reduced cost, but we have provided our patients with timely information and quality care.
>
> (88)

The results of this study are encouraging and it appears to have been rigorously conducted. It would seem that there is a need for more of this type of research to help establish the actual outcomes of patient education in a variety of settings in terms of both effect and efficiency.

Other studies have also demonstrated that suitable patient education can save costs, for example for patients nearing end-stage renal failure (Binik *et al.*, 1993), those with hypertension (Rocella and Lenfant, 1992) and for people with asthma (Liljas and Lahdensuo, 1997; Trautner *et al.*, 1993). Financial savings are, of course, only one of the potential benefits to be derived from patient education, although obviously one of the most important ones to policy makers and managers.

There are many empirical studies in which education is reported to be effective according to other outcomes. Perhaps the classic studies in this field, those of Hayward (1975), Boore (1978) and Wilson-Barnett (1978) are a good place to start. The study by Hayward examined the influence of pre-operative education for patients about their impending surgery. The results illustrated that patients did benefit from relevant pre-operative information in terms of becoming pain free, sleeping better and regaining their appetite more quickly post-operatively than the patients in the control group. This experimental design study was one of the first in nursing to examine the effect of nursing intervention upon clearly defined outcomes.

Similarly Boore (1978) examined the effect of pre-operative education on post-operative stress and recovery. This study was of an experimental design and sought to investigate whether interventions of a psychological nature (patient education) could be demonstrated physiologically through the urinary excretion of chemicals (17 hydroxycortico-steroids) which are related to the stress experienced by an individual. The greater the stress experienced the higher the excretion of the chemicals. Forty patients were in the experimental group who received pre-operative information on topics such as fasting, transfer to theatre and post-operative events and equipment. Forty patients were in the control group; they had similar contact with the researcher but the time was used for general conversation rather than for teaching. In this study it was found that the people in the experimental group did subsequently experience less stress post-operatively. Interestingly, the rate of post-operative infection in the experimental group was also less than in the control group. The results of this study serve to demonstrate that there is a link between psychological and physiological states and that patient education can be effective.

In the study reported by Wilson-Barnett (1978) the anxiety experienced by 70 patients having a barium enema and 58 having a barium meal was investigated. Subjects were divided into experimental and control groups. Those in the former group received information about their impending investigation while those in the control only received a visit from the researcher. Self-reported emotional responses were measured at four different times, ranging from before the investigation to half an hour after it. The people in the barium meal control study did not report less stress than those in the experimental group but it was pointed out that this may be a relatively less stressful event. However, for patients having a barium enema it was found that there was a significant difference in the two sets of scores. Informed patients reported that they experienced less stress than those in the control group during the x-ray. This study illustrates that providing information can alleviate anxiety. The means by which this effect is achieved were not fully understood then and they are little better understood now. However, the significance of the work lies in the fact that nurses are in a position to alleviate patient anxiety through patient education.

These three studies were innovative in their time and twenty years later still serve as useful examples of rigorous research in which the effectiveness of patient education can be examined. In the 1970s such work was rare in nursing. Fortunately, it is now rather more common and accessible.

More recent studies include that of Ferrell *et al.* (1994), who evaluated a structured pain education programme delivered in the homes of elderly patients with cancer. Sixty-six people completed the structured pain education programme covering basic pain management, pharmacological interventions and non-drug treatments. They reported that improved pain management as a result of the programme led to improved quality of life, which reflected reported improvements in physical, psychological and spiritual well-being and social concern for the people involved. They recommended that a structured rather than an informal or inconsistent approach to education should be an integral aspect of pain management.

O'Connor *et al.* (1990) investigated whether staff nurses, rather than researchers, could provide patient education which could lead to improved surgical outcomes. They followed a detailed and thorough protocol in which nurses' patient education skills were enhanced through two workshops, development of a patient education booklet and support at research and managerial levels. It was reported that:

patients who received pre-operative care from nurse subjects after the workshop experienced decreases in length of stay and use of sedatives/anti-emetics and hypnotics; these benefits did not occur or occurred to a significantly lower degree in similar patients hospitalised in a nearby control hospital.

(17)

In this study the positive value of patient education was demonstrated. However, it is important to note that the nurses were well prepared for their role. It would be unreasonable to expect nurses to educate patients if their own skills and working culture were unsuited to the work expected of them. There are many other examples of empirical research which have reported findings supportive of patient education programmes, such as those relating to patients needing coronary angioplasty (Tooth et al., 1997), cancer patients learning about radiation therapy (Poroch, 1995), people with Parkinson's Disease (Montgomery et al., 1994), patients at risk of cardiovascular disease (Bruce and Grove, 1994), people with arthritis (Fries et al., 1997; Superio-Cabuslay et al., 1996) and relating to tooth extraction (Vallerand et al., 1994).

While it is important to consider individual studies so that the details of each investigation can be appreciated, the wealth of material concerning patient education precludes consideration of all relevant work on such a basis. In such circumstances the contribution of published literature reviews is valuable. For example, in the literature review conducted by Hirano et al. (1994) they selected published studies in which education was offered to people with arthritis. The studies had to include measurement details of the variables being studied and evaluation of the education programme. Twenty-five studies met these criteria. After reviewing them to gauge the impact of the educational intervention it was suggested that an improvement in reported symptoms of people with arthritis could be achieved through patient education interventions.

Wilson-Barnett and Osborne (1983) evaluated 29 studies of patient teaching from a 'representative selection of evaluative studies' (33). They concluded that in the majority of studies there was merit in patient teaching and that nursing care should include this activity.

Some researchers have taken this approach further and conducted a re-analysis of the findings of work previously published on a particular topic, using a technique rather grandly referred to as meta-analysis (Powers and Knapp, 1990). For example, Mullen *et al.* (1992) re-analysed the results of published studies of controlled trials of cardiac patient education through the process of meta-analysis. They reported that education programmes included in their study had a quantifiable impact on blood pressure, mortality, exercise and diet. Thus through this approach they demonstrated the positive effect of education for cardiac patients. Similarly, Brown (1990) conducted a literature review and meta-analysis involving 82 experimental studies concerning the effects of patient education programmes in diabetes. She concluded that patient education did lead to an increase in patient knowledge and that it also had a positive effect upon diabetic metabolic control.

Thus over a long number of years, in a wide variety of settings and through a range of research approaches, the effectiveness of patient teaching has been reported. However, research results are not wholly supportive of the value of patient education. There are also studies available which indicate that planned programmes of patient education may not make any tangible difference to patient care. For example, Meeker (1994) investigated the effect of pre-operative education on post-operative atelectasis and the level of patient satisfaction with their education. Ninety-five patients formed the control group and forty-nine received structured education. The samples were similar but not matched. The results showed no significant difference between the two groups of patients for either outcome. However, the authors do not explain why the sample sizes were different or why they were not randomised. They do, however, acknowledge limitations to their study, which may undermine the credibility of their findings.

Ziemer (1983) reports the effects of information on post-operative coping. One hundred and eleven patients were randomly assigned to one of three groups. The first group received a five and a half minute tape-recorded message about procedures they would undergo, such as a skin prep. The second group received the same plus an explanation of the sensations they were likely to experience. Finally, those in the third group listened to the above and in addition they received taped information about coping strategies. The results of this study yielded no evidence that:

> the type of information provided for patients prior to surgery
> increased the reported frequency of coping behaviours or that
> the reported frequency of coping behaviours was related to

improved outcomes as evaluated by pain intensity, distress or selected physical complications.

(282)

The wisdom of providing patients, who were likely to be feeling stressed by the prospect of their impending surgery, with education delivered by taped messages could perhaps be questioned. Other studies have also reported only limited success for patient education programmes (Cherkin *et al.*, 1996). It must also be remembered that it is more difficult to get studies with negative or non-significant results published. Therefore there is an inherent bias in the material acquired through computerised literature searches, such as is the foundation for this book. It is likely that negative findings are under-represented.

It is important to note that not all research has supported the effectiveness of educational interventions supplied to patients. Such studies must be borne in mind and reasons why the intervention was found to be unsuccessful must be sought in order to improve the educational intervention in the future.

Do patients prefer to be educated about health problems?

The fourth reason why patient education is advocated is that patients are reported to want it and feel dissatisfied with their care if they don't receive it. Earlier in this chapter the need to consider patients'/clients' views was discussed and supported. It is therefore relevant to consider what patients say they expect or appreciate about health care. The Patients' Charter would also support this perspective (D.o.H., 1992b).

Renowned studies in this field include those of Cartwright (1964) and Raphael (1969), who reported that patients were deeply dissatisfied about the quality of communication they experienced in hospital. Reynolds (1978) reported the results of 100 interviews of surgical inpatients about the information offered regarding their treatment while in hospital. The majority (55) were not satisfied with the information received.

More recent research also supports this perspective. For example, Moser *et al.* (1993) investigated the self-perceived needs of 49 patients recovering from an acute cardiac event and compared and contrasted their views with those of their spouses. The patients and their spouses had similar needs for information although the specific details sought were different. Their need for information was ranked more highly than all other needs. Unfortunately these needs were largely unmet. For example, over 70 per cent of the sample reported that they did not receive information to prepare them to deal with an emergency.

This finding is supported by those of Smyth *et al.* (1995), who reviewed literature relating to the needs of women with breast cancer. They concluded that the women received inadequate information and support. 'Information given to patients with regard to their disease, its treatment and the impact of breast cancer on their lives, seems at best, barely adequate' (91).

The work of Bostrom *et al.* (1994) investigated the views of 76 hospital patients regarding their learning needs. The most highly prioritised needs were for information about treatment and complications, medications and subjects relating to quality of life such as how to manage pain. These items were ranked higher than, for example, community follow-up or skin care.

The researchers then conducted a second phase of the study to determine whether, at two weeks post-discharge, patients continue to rate the importance of receiving information in the same way. These needs were supported; indeed, it was found that for recently discharged patients 'the importance of most health information increases' (83).

In addition to supporting patients' expressed desire for information the authors state that their work also argues in favour of the efficiency of patient education if nurses prioritise their teaching according to expressed learning needs to make best use of the limited time available:

> As hospitals endeavour to provide the highest quality of patient care at the lowest possible cost, understanding the continuum of patient care that exists between hospital and community is critical. Ideally, nurses should strive for an 'unbroken' or 'seamless' continuum of patient care that would address patient learning needs both during and after hospitalization.
>
> (89)

Other research also supports the view that patients would like to have more information (Sengupta and Roe, 1996; Jaarsma *et al.*, 1995; Yeager *et al.*, 1995; Audit Commission, 1993).

Patient education – relevant, desirable and desired

A wide range of literature has been examined to inform the debate surrounding the above issues. The initial literature review was drawn from the large databases of Medline, BIDS and the Cumulative Index of Nursing and Allied Health Literature (CINAHLS). Key words were used and references from 1990–1998 were requested. All new references which appeared to be relevant to this book were followed up and reviewed both from the material gained during the computerised searches and from reference lists at the end of journals, books and reports. Work already known to the author was included and a small number of hand searches were also conducted. By using a wide range of material it is believed that a fair representation of the subject area is presented, although it should be acknowledged that systematic, computer-based searches will not identify all relevant work and some estimates are as low as only 50 per cent of the available material. Several older references have been included which may be regarded as classics in patient education. Students who are new to nursing may not be familiar with these works and this justifies their inclusion. Whilst it could be argued that there is no need to make a case for patient education as everyone already agrees that it is important, this situation should not be assumed. Views which seem intuitively to have value are by no means universally held, as the debate earlier in this chapter about whether patients desire participation illustrates.

This chapter has used research findings to demonstrate that patient education is relevant and important in today's changing health care environment. Moreover, it is both desirable in the sense that it appears to lead to health gain and that it is desired by many patients themselves as part of their treatment.

In the following chapter the research basis to support the process of patient education will be examined because it is imperative that practice is based on an identifiable scientific basis whenever possible. However, despite the vast amount that has been written about patient education it will be shown that not all research is sufficiently robust to enable it to be used to influence practice. Therefore research papers must be read carefully and the evidence base that we are all being urged to use in practice may be hard to find at times.

In Chapter 3 the theoretical basis for patient education will be considered. It is clearly important that we should have some understanding of the ways in which adults learn if educational interventions are to be appropriately developed and applied. Unfortunately, there is an inherent weakness in existing learning theory because it relates principally to classroom settings and is attempting to explain learning amongst people who are fit and well rather than those who are sick. There is still a great need for learning theory to be applied and tested in health care contexts and amongst patient groups.

Chapters 4 and 5 focus on the process of patient education, primarily, but not exclusively, as it takes place in hospital or in relatively acute situations. In Chapter 4 assessment of educational need and goal setting are discussed, based on research results as far as is possible, while in Chapter 5 a range of educational interventions is considered. The effectiveness of different interventions, their strengths and weaknesses and, finally, the ways in which education can be evaluated are discussed.

The vast majority of patients have a chronic rather than an acute health problem and are living in the community, therefore Chapters 6 and 7 focus on educational issues relevant to their situation and needs. In Chapter 6 several theories which purport to explain behavioural change are presented and their strengths and weaknesses discussed. The theories which are considered most relevant to the learning of cognitive information are quite different to those put forward to explain and predict learning and self-management behaviour in chronic illness situations. Building on these theories, educational interventions and issues relating specifically to the needs of people with a chronic health problem are discussed in Chapter 7. Finally, in Chapter 8 the role of nurses in patient education is examined and factors which either facilitate or hinder nurses' striving to undertake patient education are debated.

To conclude the current chapter, Kate Lorig's (1995) view of patient education in the field of rheumatology will be noted to emphasise the importance of patient education. She reminds us that there is enough research to support the view that patient education is a treatment in its own right, but it unfortunately may or may not be offered to patients, depending on local services and provision. She compares this to medication and suggests the outcry that there would be if patients were denied their medicines and tablets. Unfortunately, patients *can* be denied access to research-based patient education interventions and there is hardly any objection. This should serve to remind us all that it is time for the practice of patient education to be taken a good deal more seriously by those involved in all levels of health care.

KEY POINTS FROM CHAPTER 1

1   *The definition of patient education* adopted for use in this book
    is as follows:

> planned combinations of learning activities designed to assist
> people who are having or have had experience with illness or
> disease in making changes in their behaviour conducive to
> health.
>   (Squyres, 1980: 1 as adapted from Green, *et al.* (1980)

2   *In this book it is intended to give a broad overview of general
    issues and principles of patient education* which may be applied
    widely, rather than relate to any specific patient need or clin-
    ical condition. The book will focus on the needs of adults rather
    than children, on patients whose primary diagnosis relates to
    physical rather than mental health problems and the needs of
    patients rather than their families. The decision to exclude some
    topics was made not only to keep the book to a manageable
    size but also to be able to deal with those topics which are
    included in greater depth.

3   *Patient education is important because of the nature of disease
    and illness prevalent in our society.* As many of the health care
    problems of today relate to chronic illness and an ageing popu-
    lation the need for patient education is increased. If all health
    problems could be readily 'fixed' there would be less need for
    ongoing patient education.

4   *Patient participation is a fashionable concept in health care*
    which can only be achieved if there is adequate patient educa-
    tion. Patients should participate in their care as fully as they
    would wish to and patient education must be designed to facil-
    itate this. The notion that health professionals are in a position
    of power over patients needs to be revised, and if possible we
    should aim for a situation in which patients and health profes-
    sionals have equal power. Only then can patients be considered
    as partners in the educative process. However, not all patients
    want to participate actively in their care and it is important
    that individuals' preferences are sought and not assumed. The
    frameworks for participation developed by Szasz and Hollender
    (1956) or Roter (1987) are thought to be useful guides to

practice, illustrating that patients' roles are dynamic rather than static.

5   *Patient education is an effective intervention* in a wide variety of settings. Research was included to indicate that educating patients can contribute to the provision of an effective and efficient service and that it does not lead to unnecessary expense. However, it was also mentioned that not all patient education interventions lead to the desired outcomes.

6   *Patients wish to be educated.* If a holistic service, designed to satisfy patients, is to be provided, patient education must be included. Education is an integral part of treatment. It should therefore be considered as deserving of as much attention as other elements of care.

Chapter 2

Investigating education: research issues

Introduction

Since at least the early 1970s, there have been repeated calls for a sound research base to inform clinical practice. These calls have been going on for even longer in America. However, a substantial problem concerns the lack of suitable research to provide such a base. There are plenty of research reports for nurses to read, but these are not necessarily all examples of rigorous research. In this chapter, potential limitations in the available research into patient education will be discussed, with the aim of helping nurses get to grips with the importance of adopting a critical stance when choosing studies to inform practice. The desire for nursing to be evidence-based presumes that we have an adequate body of evidence upon which to base nursing practice. Unfortunately, weaknesses in research design undermine the value of reported results, which in turn erode the value of the 'evidence'. As will be shown in this chapter, research-based evidence may not always be available. This does not mean that the *need* for evidence-based practice is undermined, just that the evidence may be in short supply. Alternative sources of evidence will be mentioned and the implications of *not* using research to underpin patient education will also be briefly considered.

The importance of a scientific basis for patient/client education

The current emphasis in the United Kingdom on evidence-based health care requires that medical and non-medical professionals ensure that their clinical practice is founded on scientifically derived findings rather than on intuition and ritual.

(Hicks and Hennessy, 1997: 595)

As long ago as 1979, James Smith attempted to clarify whether the practice of nursing is based on a body of knowledge developed from systematic investigation (J. Smith, 1979). He noted that there were two important aspects to this issue: first, there was little high quality research available for practitioners to use; and, second, it was difficult to put what research there was into daily practice. Furthermore, if research was used it was very difficult to estimate its effect, since nursing care was not usually evaluated in a systematic and thorough way. Fortunately, some changes have occurred since Smith was noting these problems. Not only is there much more research available, but nurses in general are more aware of the need to use it in practice. Furthermore, in some areas, such as nurse development units, it may be possible to evaluate the outcomes of care in a tangible way. However, it could also be argued that the issues identified by Smith nearly twenty years ago are still influencing care today. The work of Mike Walsh and Pauline Ford (1989; 1992) and Walshe *et al.* (1995) to name but a few, suggests that care is not usually research-based.

Even so, the culture in which care is delivered has changed and this changing culture now adds weight to the case for research-based practice in nursing. In future, the funding of care will be influenced by the extent to which it can be demonstrated to be science-based and to have a positive effect on patient outcomes:

> The current ideology of open accounting, cost effectiveness, efficiency targets and audit means that it is no longer acceptable to deliver care that cannot be justified on proper empirical grounds.
>
> (Hicks and Hennessy, 1997: 595)

This trend is likely to gather strength. For example, as Regan (1998) reports, both the NHS Executive and the Royal College of Nursing launched major clinical effectiveness initiatives in 1996 with the aim of promoting evidence-based practice across the nation. The ultimate intention is that all people with a particular condition should receive the same form of care, based on a rationale which can be defended by evidence from strictly controlled research conditions.

Thus, the term *evidence-based practice* is currently in fashion. It includes research-based evidence, but other forms of evidence, such as expert opinion, can also be used to support interventions. However, the most powerful way in which nurses can demonstrate that nursing is evidence-based is by means of research, although whether or not research-based care equates to clinical effectiveness has yet to be established (Regan, 1998).

Research and patient education

It has been noted that future funding of care is likely to be related to the ability of proponents of particular interventions to demonstrate that these interventions are research-based and effective. The education of patients is itself an intervention, and, because of the staff time and resources it consumes, has a cost, and, therefore, funding implications. This chapter focuses on the quality of the research which is available to underpin patient education. Clearly, nurses should not base practice upon flawed research, yet the availability of research which is sufficiently rigorous to be worth applying in practice may be limited (Hunter, 1996). Indeed, with reference to patient education, the work of Brown (1990) and others (O'Halloran and Altmaier, 1995) demonstrates that the theoretical basis for patient education may not be as sound as we would wish. Some of the weaknesses which may adversely influence research in patient education will now be considered.

Reading the literature – issues which compromise the quality of research

In order to make an objective appraisal of a piece of research it is recommended that a systematic critique of the material is conducted. As Duffy (1985: 539) has commented:

> We must learn to sort through what is weak and what is strong in our colleagues' work to be able to apply it to practice.

Duffy points out that when judging research we are looking at the research process itself, not only the reported findings, in order to decide whether the work is credible or not. Different criteria have been developed for going about this critical appraisal (Ganong, 1987; Droogan and Song, 1996). The checklist which Duffy developed was applied by Brown (1990) to evaluate the quality of reported research into education of patients with diabetes. Fortyseven studies, available from 1954 to 1986, met Brown's inclusion criteria. Twenty-nine (62 per cent) had been published as journal articles and the other 18 studies (38 per cent) were unpublished, in the form of research theses or reports. She found considerable limitations in the patient education studies reviewed, including:

- lack of definition of the variables being investigated
- no operational definitions
- lack of identification of research questions
- inadequate reporting of the development and content of instruments (e.g. questionnaires) used
- inadequate reporting of sampling (how were people selected, what population were they drawn from?)
- drop out rates (attrition) from some studies not explained
- clear description of the teaching intervention omitted (who did the teaching, in what way and how long after teaching was the outcome evaluated?).

Although Brown's (1990) work focused on the education of people with diabetes, it serves to illustrate that not all published material should necessarily be considered valid. Using Brown's findings as a framework, some of the problems caused by weaknesses in the research process as it applies to patient education will now be explored. The ability to select rigorously conducted work upon which to base teaching is an important skill if practice is to be based on a sound empirical foundation, and readers may wish to consider the issues debated below in some detail, and to apply them when examining the research literature as it applies to education in their own fields of work.

Research approach

A *paradigm* is a way of looking at an issue, and involves more than just the design of a study or the methods used, including instead an individual's whole philosophical approach to the inquiry (Polit and Hungler, 1995). The term is relevant when considering research to investigate patient education, because the paradigm used will reflect the researcher's way of conceptualising the issue. The two main research paradigms are *quantitative* and *qualitative* approaches and the merits and weaknesses of each of these general approaches are widely debated amongst nursing researchers.

Quantitative research is concerned with 'precise measurement, replicability, prediction and control' (Powers and Knapp, 1990:

120). Thus, a quantitative approach to education may focus on knowledge or skills acquired after a teaching session. Steps will be made to measure knowledge before and after the teaching and the amount of knowledge will be translated into numbers. These numbers might then be used as indicators of knowledge gained.

It is generally proposed that a quantitative approach is most suited to research into the physical sciences, where the research environment can be strictly controlled and experimental studies can be conducted. The belief that such research is thoroughly controlled has led to its being referred to as 'hard' research (Polit and Hungler, 1995) and it has the aura of being an objective and scientific method of investigation (Williams et al., 1988). However, this premise has been challenged (Webb, 1992). For example, Berg (1989) has suggested that there is a tendency to associate science with numbers and precision, but as will be discussed below it can be misleading to assume that numbers are necessarily accurate.

Qualitative research is an alternative approach to inquiry. It covers a wide range of research designs and methods, but in essence it refers to organising and interpreting non-numerical data such as individuals' own words, conversations or behaviours to discover important underlying dimensions, patterns, themes and relationships (Polit and Hungler, 1995).

Those who wish to support qualitative approaches could argue that patient education is too complex a phenomenon to be reduced to a set of numbers and that other vital components of the educational process could be excluded when controlling a research situation. Thus it could not be argued that a complex subject such as patient education may not be fully revealed through quantitative methods and an approach which allows for the influence and inter-dependence of many aspects of people and their environment may be needed to promote understanding (Streubert and Carpenter, 1995; Dzurec, 1990). Research regarding people may be more fruitfully conducted by applying a more holistic method of investigation in which the totality of an experience or a situation is investigated (Benoliel, 1984; Polit and Hungler, 1995; Hicks and Hennessy, 1997).

As people are the focus of investigations in the social sciences, it is often impossible to control the research environment. The elements of interest may be intangible and perhaps not amenable to investigation in isolation from their social context (Streubert and Carpenter, 1995). For example, in patient education the actual content of a teaching session will not be the only influence on the patient and it may be inappropriate to assume that there is a linear relationship between teaching and patient knowledge. Personality, previous experience or social circumstances, for example, may all influence how much a person will learn and it could be argued that education must be considered holistically rather than in a highly selective (some may say reductionist) fashion.

According to Berg (1989: 6) qualitative techniques 'provide a means of assessing unquantifiable facts about the actual people researchers observe and talk to'. Nyhlin (1990) goes further, and suggests that phenomena in the social world cannot be explained in a scientific quantitative way.

Choice of investigative method may be controversial at times. Both qualitative and quantitative approaches are valuable and the most appropriate way to select an approach is to do this with sensitivity to the kinds of research question being addressed. In a broad sense qualitative inquiry can help our understanding of needs and experiences. If an insight into the learning experience of an individual is required it may be more suitable to use a qualitative approach. However, qualitative research is limited in that it is not amenable to powerful statistical analysis (Berg, 1989). It enables description rather than testing of ideas.

In contrast, quantitative methods, when appropriately applied, allow defined variables to be measured, statistical analysis to be undertaken and cause and effect relationships to be tested. This form of analysis is essential to furthering the knowledge base of a discipline. For example, if the effect of an educational intervention is to be evaluated, a quantitative design would usually be selected. In a review such as Brown's (1990) the studies are largely quantitative and the criteria she employs relate strongly to a quantitative paradigm.

It is also possible to use more than one research approach to a particular problem (Cormack, 1996) and blend qualitative and quantitative methods. For example, after critically analysing the place of experimental research in the development of nursing knowledge, Wilson-Barnett (1991) suggested that a combination of approaches might be a valuable option. In this way it could be possible to gain from the power afforded by statistical analysis of quantitative data and yet also have the richness of qualitative findings.

However it should not be assumed that combining approaches in itself is good. The purpose of the technique and the way in which multiple sources of the data are used to enhance the completeness of the study must be made explicit (Knafl and Breitmayer, 1991). The use of any particular approach to an investigation is influenced by the nature of the problem to be investigated, and the allegiance which the researcher has to a particular paradigm (Cohen and Manion, 1980; Morse and Field, 1996; Berg, 1989).

In reading research reports, it is wise to consider whether the research approach adopted is appropriate to answering the question the researcher claims to be investigating. For example, it may be felt that adopting a quantitative approach to the examination of the in-depth experiences of individuals involved in an educational programme is inappropriate, whilst the use of a qualitative method to examine cause and effect relationships (for example, the effect of a teaching programme on patient adherence to medication) may be considered equally inappropriate. The researcher may be able to offer an acceptable rationale for the use of these techniques, but the reader will want to be sure that this rationale is sufficiently robust to allow us to have confidence in the validity of the report's findings and their relevance to patient education in clinical practice.

Clear definition of purpose and variables

Brown (1990: 56) noted that variables were frequently referred to without definition:

> For example, the purpose of the study may have been to measure 'accuracy' or 'control' as an outcome of a diabetes teaching programme; however, authors never defined accuracy or control, either conceptually or operationally.

It is important that the concepts of interest are clearly defined. If they are not then there will be ambiguity about what was actually being investigated. As a result, the outcomes will also be unclear and future researchers will not be able to replicate the study should they wish to. For example, Greenfield et al. (1985) noted a lack of agreement among researchers in the area of 'patient participation' in care. If a study were designed to test whether an educational intervention helped patients to participate more actively in care, without clearly defining what 'active participation' meant for the purposes of the study, readers might find it hard to judge the true impact of the intervention. Furthermore, it might not be possible to compare the results of a study which lacked clear definition with those from other investigations because readers would not know whether they were comparing 'like with like'.

Similarly, the purpose of the research (research questions/hypotheses) must be clearly stated so that the reader of the report is able to comprehend fully what the researchers set out to achieve. As Bear and Moody (1990: 147) have suggested: 'Fuzzy thinking at this early stage of the research process will obstruct the success of the research project.' If definitions and research purpose are not clearly stated in the report it is not subsequently possible to evaluate whether stated aims and objectives have been fulfilled. As with the general research approach, inappropriate or inadequate definition of purpose and variables in the study undermine our confidence in the applicability of the supposed findings to patient education.

Sampling

Sampling is the process of recruiting people to take part in an investigation. For example, if a nurse wished to evaluate the effect that a teaching package had on stoma patients it would not be possible to include all people with a stoma in the study. Therefore a selection or a subset of this population of people with stomas is taken, and forms the sample. How the selection is made will have an impact on the results of the study. Sampling procedures are included in all standard research texts (Parahoo, 1997; Cormack, 1996) and will not be described here. However, the influence that inadequate sampling has on subsequent results will be outlined.

According to Duffy (1985: 543), when evaluating the adequacy of a sample, it is important that the

- subject population (sampling frame) is described
- sampling method is described
- sampling method is justified – especially if a convenience sample is used rather than a random sample
- sample size is sufficient to enable appropriate statistical analysis to be undertaken
- possible sources of sampling error are identified (as these could lead to bias in the results)
- standards for protection of subjects are discussed

When applying Duffy's criteria to research on patient education, Brown (1990) found that:

Sampling methods were diverse; however, authors did not specify their exact sampling procedures or describe the population from which the sample was taken. Generally, most samples were convenience samples obtained from . . . persons attending clinics or residing on inpatient hospital units.

(56)

This finding raises several important points. If different studies use different types of sampling, it can be hard to compare and contrast the findings of one study with those of another. In the same way, if studies produce conflicting results it may be difficult to determine whether the differences were due to the teaching intervention itself or to the fact that the samples selected were themselves different. If the method of sampling is not included in the report at all, then the reader cannot comment upon the adequacy or appropriateness of the method. Similarly if the population from which the sample is drawn is not clearly stated, it is not possible to decide how adequately the population is represented.

Thus if a research study reports the success of an educational intervention it is important that readers know how many patients were involved in the study. Were they a few, ideal, hand-picked subjects or could the patients involved be considered as regular, typical, average, representatives of the larger patient group.

Convenience samples are frequently used in nursing research, literally selecting people who are conveniently available to the researcher. However, this method of sampling does place limitations upon the research. If samples are drawn for convenience it is not possible to know whether they are in some way biased. Are the people who agree to participate in a research study different to those who do not? Are they more interested in their condition and care, and more likely to follow treatment than those who do not? When the results are presented it is more difficult to apply them to the wider population due to the risk of unknown bias (Newell, 1996). When results based on a convenience sample are presented it must be remembered that the sample used may not adequately represent the total population.

If the method of sampling is adequate, a larger sample is likely to be more representative of the population than a smaller one. Unfortunately, in nursing, samples tend to be small. Smith (1994) reviewed the quality of nursing research (in general rather than educational specifically) and noted that nursing studies tend to use small samples (25–200 range) and these are usually recruited by convenience sampling methods. Furthermore, many statistical tests are based upon the principle of using a random sample (Thomas, 1990). If such tests are applied to a convenience sample the results may not be valid.

The attrition rate (that is, the drop-out rate) should also be reported in studies which claim to evaluate patient education. If the impact of education is to be measured over time, for example, to find out how memorable or influential the education has been, it is relevant to know how many patients were still involved at the completion of the study and how many had 'dropped out'. It may be expected that the longer the teaching intervention and the longer the follow-up period the greater the expected attrition rate might be. Moreover, participants who drop out might well be quite different from those who continue to the end of the study. If the attrition rate was high, we should be less inclined to regard the remaining participants as representative of either the original sample or the population from which it was drawn. Thus, the reader needs to know the proportion of people who withdrew from the study. Imagine if you were interested in applying a reported teaching strategy, would you still be interested if you found out that most patients had dropped out before the intervention was completed?

No attempt has been made in this section to cover comprehensively the subject of sampling. The aim has been to stress that there must be a rationale and rigour when selecting subjects for both qualitative and quantitative studies. When reading research about patient education, the adequacy of the sample must be considered. In order to do this, issues of sampling must be sufficiently well described within the research reports to allow us to assess their acceptability. As Oldham (1996: 3) has commented: 'All too often samples are too small, or are unreliable and not valid, rendering the results from otherwise carefully designed studies meaningless.'

Describing the educational intervention

Brown (1990) reports that a clear description of the educational intervention is often missing in studies of patient education. If nurses are reading a research article in the hope that it could be applied to their own area of practice, then details of the way in which the teaching was undertaken, by whom and for how long, need to be included. Without such information it is difficult to judge the adequacy of an intervention. If an intervention required large resources – was intensive on staff time for example – it might indicate to the reader that it would not be feasible to apply it to their own area.

O'Halloran and Altmaier (1995) reviewed research designed to evaluate educational preparation for adults about to undergo surgery or an invasive medical procedure. They hoped to clarify 'what intervention is most appropriate to which patients?' which is crucial if the most valuable interventions are to be applied in practice. Unfortunately, they found it was not possible to answer this question. One of the reasons why they could not answer it was that 'similarly named interventions can be implemented very differently. Thus, overall conclusions of effectiveness must be drawn with some caution' (10).

Unfortunately, O'Halloran and Altmaier do not report their own methodology (other than that it is a review): they fail to give details of how they searched for studies, whether all studies were included, whether inclusion/exclusion criteria were applied and if so what they were, and they do not state the overall number of studies in their review. These omissions subsequently limit the value of their own work.

Measuring the outcomes of patient education

In order to judge whether a teaching initiative has had any effect it is important to identify the outcomes of the educational intervention and how they can be measured. The desired outcome of an educational intervention can be:

- *psychomotor*, such as a planned change in behaviour or the acquisition of a skill
- *cognitive*, such as knowledge gain
- *affective*, concerning attitudes, values and beliefs

Psychomotor outcomes

With care, psychomotor skills can be directly observed and thus they are amenable to measurement, although this is not as easy to do accurately as may be assumed (Caron, 1985; Cramer and Spilker, 1991).

In Chapter 1, it was stated that the purpose of patient education is to help people to make changes in their behaviour which are likely to improve their health. If the ultimate goal is behavioural, then education will need to be evaluated using behavioural (psychomotor) criteria. Whilst individuals can be asked directly about their behaviour, a more accurate approach in a research setting is to observe, and 'capture' or measure, the behaviour. The practical implications of this are obvious, as we are not usually at liberty to watch people for prolonged periods of time. For example, we are unlikely to be able to check whether, after an educational intervention, people have changed their diet, stopped smoking, increased exercise, taken their tablets, used their inhalers or practised safe sex. As you might expect, behaviour may also change simply because individuals are aware they are being observed (Parahoo, 1997).

Various methods and techniques can be used to make the recording of psychomotor or behavioural variables reliable and valid and these are not covered here (see Cramer and Spilker, 1991; Polit and Hungler, 1995). However, when judging the value of a research report which claims that behavioural change was achieved as a result of a teaching intervention the reader must consider if the method by which behavioural change was defined and measured was valid.

Cognitive and affective outcomes

Cognitive and affective variables such as knowledge or beliefs are intangible, and so cannot be observed directly. They can, however, be indicated indirectly by means of instruments designed for the purpose. As Bradley (1994) has pointed out, people who have limited experience with instrument design will be tempted to use ready-made ones because it takes much less skill merely to administer them: 'there is a danger that off-the-peg scales are overused and misused in inappropriate circumstances because they are readily available, inexpensive and easy and the user does not stop to ask "Is it appropriate for my purposes?"' (8).

In the case of a research study to evaluate the impact of teaching to increase knowledge or alter health beliefs, it is crucially important that the measurement instruments can measure these variables. The review and analysis by Brown (1990) led her to comment: 'Measurement of knowledge was one of the most seriously flawed outcome variables in the sample of studies included in this analysis' (57).

The measurement instruments most frequently used to measure abstract variables are questionnaires and attitude scales. These instruments form the link between what is observable (the respondent's scores) and the unobservable variables – for example, knowledge. The accuracy with which instruments can measure these variables is conventionally discussed in terms of validity and reliability. According to Carmines (1986: 23):

> Many of the most important variables in the social sciences cannot be directly observed. As a consequence they can only be measured indirectly through the use . . . of measured indicators that represent the (unseen) variables. . . . The fundamental question with regard to measurement inferences is how validly and reliably these indicators represent the unobserved theoretical constructs.

Unfortunately, literature indicates that this is an area which is frequently overlooked in nursing research (Thomas, 1990; Deane, 1991; Goodwin and Goodwin, 1991).

Reliability and validity of instruments used in educational research

Thus, if in a research article it is claimed that patients knew more, or felt different about some aspect of health care, after a teaching intervention it stands to reason that the instrument used to measure 'knowledge gain' or 'attitude change' must be accurate. This is no different from the way in which we would expect a physical parameter such as blood pressure or a blood level to be measured using a suitable, accurate instrument. While this sounds like common sense it is interesting to learn that the instruments used to measure educational outcomes are often inaccurate.

In the study by Brown (1990) previously cited, it was reported that:

> The major limitation of many studies related to lack of instrument reliability and validity, particularly in knowledge and skill areas.
>
> (56)

The reliability of the data-gathering tools is an important criterion which must be established if research results are to be meaningful. However, even in the physical sciences it is not possible to obtain perfectly reliable measures. In the social sciences, the situation is made more complicated because it is often necessary to measure abstract concepts such as health beliefs or attitudes. None the less, the need for reliable and valid measurement remains crucial.

As it is acknowledged that the instruments will not be entirely reliable, it must be accepted that results will always be influenced to some degree by measurement error. The amount of error generated through the use of measurement tools affects the accuracy of the reported results. Thus it is vital that authors report the reliability of any instruments used in their research to enable readers to evaluate the credibility they attach to the reported results.

Validity is vital if results of a study are to have meaning. Validity may be defined as 'The degree to which an instrument measures what it is intended to measure' (Polit and Hungler, 1995: 656). So if a study sets out to investigate whether an educational intervention leads to a reduction in, say, anxiety, then the instrument must measure 'anxiety' and not some other psychological variable such as stress or depression; just as when a biotechnologist develops a test to measure urea the instrument must measure urea and not some other chemical. Estimating validity is therefore about assessing the extent to which an instrument measures what it claims to measure. There are three main types of validity, content, construct and criterion related, and of these construct validity is considered the most important (Deane, 1991).

According to Stenner et al.:

> The process of ascribing meaning to scores produced by a measurement procedure is generally recognized as the most important task in developing an educational or psychological measure, be it an achievement test . . . or personality scale . . . this process . . . is commonly referred to as construct validation.
>
> (1983: 305)

Whilst it is vital that these properties are investigated, it has been noted by Goodwin and Goodwin (1991) that there appears to be a lack of attention given to instrument design in nursing:

> Given the very abstract nature of many of the variables that we want to measure, the largely limited consideration of construct validity is especially distressing.
>
> (235)

Nunnally (1981) offers a more basic way of considering the issue:

One could rightly argue that all this fuss and bother about construct validity really boils down to something rather home-spun – namely, circumstantial evidence for the usefulness of a new measurement method. New measurement methods, like most new ways of doing things, should not be trusted until they have proved themselves in many applications.

(109)

The means by which validity may be estimated are described in a number of standard texts (Parahoo, 1997; Polit and Hungler, 1995). It is important that practitioners involved in patient education who are striving to use research to deliver evidence-based practice are aware that validity is a crucial issue which must be commented on in a research report. If validity is either not reported, or is said to be limited, then the reader must interpret results with caution.

Validity and reliability in qualitative research

As the paradigm underlying qualitative research is fundamentally different from quantitative research the same criteria cannot be used to judge the quality of qualitative work. Measurement is not the goal of qualitative methods; they focus upon the:

> extent to which the data provides insights, knowledge and understandings of the meanings, attributes, characteristics and/ or lifeways of people under study.
>
> (Leininger, 1987: 34)

One of the major constraints upon the reliability of qualitative research is the difficulty in replicating qualitative data because the research setting is not controlled. As human behaviour is never static the study cannot be exactly replicated, regardless of methods or design (LeCompte and Goetz, 1982).

Although it may be difficult to establish the reliability of quali-tative work, one of its strengths is that it may generate the most valid of any data which attempts to give a realistic view of the informant's world. This is so because individual responses may be recorded fully, directly and often verbatim, rather than trying to equate a complex response to a single number.

The goals and methods of investigation in qualitative research have led to it being considered a less valid approach by some people

(Clarke, 1992). Indeed, 'a common criticism directed at so-called qualitative investigation is that it fails to adhere to canons of reliability and validity' (LeCompte and Goetz, 1982: 31). However this is so because the remit of the research is different, thus the criteria for estimating credibility and rigour in qualitative studies are also different (Leininger, 1987; LeCompte and Goetz, 1982). The means by which credibility of data may be estimated are available elsewhere (Streubert and Carpenter, 1995).

Whilst it is important to be aware that considerations of reliability and validity vary according to the approach used, it is always vital to conduct an investigation with rigour. The criteria and methods used to examine the credibility of research findings must be included in the research report. In this way, the reader has the opportunity to assess how far the conventions regarding reliability and validity have been followed in the study being reported. Important breaches of these conventions will limit the extent to which we will wish either to be confident of the report's findings or to use them to guide our approaches to patient education.

Conclusion to issues compromising the quality of research

The above section is not a complete critique of the research process applied to patient education research. Rather, it has taken the findings of Brown (1990) and used them as a framework to consider commonly found limitations in educational research. This framework is recommended for use by the student or clinician faced with the task of assessing the quality of studies which purport to investigate patient education. It may well be that studies investigated contain so many conceptual and methodological flaws that it is impossible to draw any meaningful conclusions from them. The findings of such studies should, of course, then never find their way into clinical practice. By contrast, a study which demonstrates very few such flaws is likely to be robust and, in consequence, to convince us of the arguments its findings seek to support. Fortunately, this latter category of studies is apparently on the increase, and Brown (1990) has observed that the quality of research reports is improving with time, indicating we are becoming increasingly skilled in educational research methods.

This work of Brown's is supported by more recent reports, of a more general nature, illustrating that evidence-based practice is called for but that the evidence may be hard to find (Hunter, 1996; Griffiths, 1995). Yvonne Moores (1997), Chief Nursing Officer, also draws attention to this issue:

Nurses . . . frequently lack the required sound evidence of the potential effectiveness of intervention. We are frequently unable to define or measure health outcome. This would enable us to know what we should be doing and how we can implement knowledge into practice.

(3)

Without appropriate evidence Hicks and Hennessy (1997) warn that:

it is conceivable that those areas of clinical practice that cannot be subjected to the experimental paradigm will not enjoy empirical substantiation and therefore will continue to be rooted in hunch, prejudice and supposition.

(597)

This view can be applied more widely. If practitioners cannot avail themselves of good quality research of any sort, the consequence is likely, of necessity, to be practice which is not, and cannot be, based on rigorously produced evidence.

Walshe et al. (1995) suggest that the 'rhetoric of evidence-based medicine will outpace the realities of clinical practice' (29). The same problem is likely to apply to nursing. If nursing practice is not research-based, what is the alternative?

The alternatives to a scientific approach

The perspective which will be adopted throughout this text is that nursing practice should be research-based as far as is possible. However, it is acknowledged that there are ways of knowing which are not derived from empirical scientific inquiry. For example, Carper (1978: 14) suggests that there are four fundamental patterns of knowing in nursing:

1   empirics, the science of nursing
2   aesthetics, the art of nursing
3   personal knowing, how well we know ourselves
4   ethics, the component of moral knowledge in nursing

Only the first is based on scientific research. The second, the art of nursing, is also highly relevant in patient education because the manner in which patient education is conducted involves art. Art in nursing may be thought of as the 'dimension which adds quality to technical proficiency' (Holmes, 1991: 445). This suggests that, knowing all the latest facts and details and offering them to a patient, in itself may not make a teaching session effective. In addition it is all the experience, communication skills, understanding of individuals' needs and many other attributes of nurses themselves, which are drawn together and applied during patient education which will determine the success or failure of a teaching intervention. O'Brien (1990) (cited by Gray and Pratt (1991: 4)) has suggested that artistry in nursing can be 'equated with the ability of nurses to view patients holistically and adapt their skill base to serve individual needs'. This draws in the concepts of expertise and intuition, qualities which nurses bring to bear in individual situations, which can make patient education an individualised experience rather than something which could be applied by a robot. These are important dimensions of educational interventions and must not be overlooked. However, art or aesthetics is not yet sufficiently understood for it to stand on its own as 'evidence' upon which to base practice. The same could be said of personal knowing and ethics: they also have a part to play in patient education, and contribute to ways of knowing in nursing but do not constitute evidence to the same extent as scientifically generated knowledge.

Vaughan (1992) suggests there are three main ways of gaining knowledge. First, what she terms tenacity, following convention: 'I know about this because it has always been like this and I will accept it as being true.' Moody (1990: 20) refers to this form of knowledge: 'as folklore, conventional wisdom or the common stock of knowledge'. Second, knowledge can be gained from a person in authority or an expert. The status of such people may have been gained through various routes such as study, experience or role modelling. This way of knowing has recently received considerable attention in nursing, for example from Benner (1984), Meerabeau (1992) and Carnevali and Thomas (1993). Third, she suggests *a priori* knowledge which is derived from logical deduction. Evidence comes from other sources such as television, books, public opinion, which an individual's own reasoning processes accept as legitimate sources. In this way people can know of things indirectly.

However, these ways of knowing are of unproven accuracy. Their value will depend upon the legitimacy of the sources of knowledge.

Ultimately these forms of knowing place the learner in the position of deciding whether to accept the knowledge or not. Yet learners may not be able to discern between legitimate and unacceptable sources. Whilst there are ways in which research-based knowledge can be critically examined it is more difficult to scrutinise other sources of knowledge. It is the transparency of research-generated knowledge that deems it a more powerful source:

> Traditionally, the scientific process has been considered a superior method of knowing, in that knowledge is derived through systematic observation of empirical data (empirics) to validate a proposition or hypothesis, thus providing for greater control for errors in judgement.
>
> (Moody, 1990: 30)

It is through research that nursing has the greatest chance of developing professional status. In the arena of patient education we must be able to demonstrate that we are using a rational, evidence-based approach if patient education is to be viewed as a professional activity. If nurses use conventional wisdom, as was mentioned above, as a basis for patient education, it could be argued that it is based on subjective views and perspectives which would not stand scrutiny with any other discipline (Ford and Walsh, 1994).

Clearly, in a health service culture calling for evidence-based practice such an approach to patient education could not be endorsed. Similarly, practice according to ritual actions is difficult to justify, although this has been attempted (Biley and Wright, 1997). According to Walsh and Ford (1989: ix):

> Ritual action implies carrying out a task without thinking it through in a problem solving, logical way. The nurse does something because this is the way it has always been done. Perhaps ... 'This is the way Sister likes it done'.

For example, a pre-operative teaching schedule which is delivered in a standardised way to all patients the night before, or the morning of, surgery as a matter of routine, regardless of individual needs or evidence of effect can no longer be condoned, even if it is a hallowed part of institutional life.

It has been argued by Hendricks and Baume (1997) that nursing is not adequately recompensed for the work that it delivers and that too small a proportion of the health care budget is allocated to nursing. It is argued here that nursing will only be able to demand greater reimbursement if it can demonstrate that it does not operate according to conventional wisdom or ritual, but that there is a credible research base for practice and nurses can demonstrate that what they do has a valuable outcome. Although, as Antrobus (1997) quite rightly reminds us, it will never be possible to capture all that nurses do using quantitative methods.

Conclusion

In this chapter the case has been made that patient education must be guided by research findings. At the same time it is suggested that research on this topic must be selected with care as it has been demonstrated that research may have significant limitations. Some of the main weaknesses, as described by Brown (1990), have been discussed with the aim of heightening awareness of the need for caution when reading published reports. Thus we have a paradox. On the one hand we are urged to indulge only in practice which can be said to be evidence-based, with, preferably, evidence derived from quantitative research methods. Yet, in this chapter it has been suggested that many studies concerning patient education do not stand scrutiny. How can we deliver evidence-based practice when we lack vital evidence? Clearly one way forward is to attempt to discriminate between robust and weak research evidence, and a considerable part of this chapter has described several criteria which we may use to help inform this discriminatory process.

Other ways of knowing surely have a contribution to make to nursing, and when the potential weaknesses of quantitatively derived results are taken into account, other evidence such as expert opinion or intuition, may not be as inferior as some may claim. None the less other forms of evidence do not yet carry the same credibility as empirically-based knowledge. Least defensible of all the alternatives is basing practice on conventional wisdom or ritual action. Such practice is unlikely to extend our understanding of patient education and is equally unlikely to benefit patients.

In the next six chapters of this book, theory and research, from a variety of disciplines, relating to patient education will be discussed with the aim of teasing out points for good practice. While accepting that research must be read with care, it is acknowledged that there are also examples of good research which can be used to inform practice. What can be particularly useful is where several authors develop an area of research on a particular topic or theme which generate findings which support each other and thus help to increase the credibility of each individual study.

Research investigations which have identified problems and inadequacies in patient education will be presented to emphasise the importance of, and need for, providing high quality patient education. Theory, strategies, protocols and initiatives which have been found to enhance patient education will be suggested. In this book, published research findings drawn from a variety of respected sources will be drawn together. The aim of all this is to help other nurses to identify studies or principles about patient education which may be usefully applied, and preferably tested, in their own area of work.

KEY POINTS FROM CHAPTER TWO

1   *The current health care culture* is driving home the need for nursing interventions which can be justified and defended. Ideally nursing should be an evidence-based profession and, preferably, evidence should be borne of rigorous research.

2   *Analysis of literature on patient education illustrates that it cannot be assumed that all published research is of a high standard.* Therefore, readers and potential consumers of research need to read research reports critically and objectively.

3   Using a report by Sharon Brown (1990) as a framework, *key factors which have been found to influence the quality of research* are presented. This framework can be used as a set of criteria according to which the credibility (or otherwise) of published research reports may be judged.

4   *A research approach appropriate* to the research questions being investigated should be used.

5   *A clear definition* of the purpose of the study and variables should be included.

6   *Sampling* techniques should be clearly explained and justified.

7   The *educational intervention should be clearly described* so that readers can understand exactly what was done.

8   *The outcomes of the educational intervention* must be defined and measured accurately so that the impact of the intervention can be evaluated.

9   *Other forms of evidence* upon which to base practice include expert opinion or intuition, and, in the absence of empirical evidence, these may be used to justify educational interventions.

10 *Least defensible of all is basing practice on conventional wisdom* or ritual action. Such practice is unlikely to extend our understanding of patient education and is unlikely to benefit patients.

Chapter 3

Learning theories as a basis for patient education

Introduction

Research, theory and practice are closely entwined. In the previous chapter research issues relating to patient education were examined. In this chapter theory relating to the education of adults will be discussed, while the focus of the next two chapters will be the practice of patient education. In reality these three areas are not independent of each other. The interdependence of research, theory and practice has been likened to a three-legged stool. If any one of the three legs is missing the entire stool becomes useless. Similarly, if nursing does not strive to unite research, theory and practice, resultant nursing activity will be less effective.

There are sufficient studies available to indicate that patient education can make a positive contribution to patients' quality of life and that it must be considered a vital part of care (Hathaway, 1986; Lindeman, 1988; O'Connor et al., 1990; Brown, 1990; Roach et al., 1995). Yet we also know that not all patients are satisfied with the information they receive (Audit Commission, 1993; Moser et al., 1993; Smyth et al., 1995). Moreover, we are not yet confident about how patients learn and which teaching strategies are most appropriate to particular people and situations. We do not yet have a sufficiently developed scientific basis for patient education. Patient education should not be based on a trial and error approach to selection of interventions, but until we have a good understanding of how people learn we cannot really hope to fulfil their learning needs in an objective manner.

Learning theories and the concept of adult education known as andragogy will be discussed in this chapter in order to help clarify their relevance to patient education. The way in which knowledge of theory can influence assessment of patients and selection of teaching strategies will also be considered.

Learning theories

Theory is useful as it offers an explanation of reality (Sims, 1991). If we can understand how adults learn then we have a better opportunity to provide valuable and successful education. If we do not understand how patients learn how can we hope to provide effective teaching for them? According to Barnum (1990: 1) a theory is a 'statement that purports to account for or characterize some phenomenon'. Therefore, a theory of learning should account for or characterise the way in which people learn. As such it should be relevant to promoting our understanding of learning and how learning can be enhanced. A theory is more specific than a model and while a theory, when sufficiently tested, can contribute to science, a theory does not constitute science. Fawcett (1992) suggests that science is the rigorous research activity involved in the testing of theories in practice using systematic, controlled, and analytical activity. Such work helps advance our knowledge. We do not yet have a particular theory to underpin patient education but there are many theories of learning developed in the disciplines of education and psychology, and by testing existing theory in practice settings nurses can contribute to the development of a scientific basis for patient education.

There are theories of learning and theories of teaching and both are important. Knowles (1990) clarifies the differences by citing Gagne (1972: 56):

> A distinction can be made between theories of learning and theories of teaching. While theories of learning deal with the ways in which an organism learns, theories of teaching deal with the ways in which a person influences an organism to learn.

Knowles goes on to state that 'Presumably, the learning theory subscribed to by a teacher will influence his theory of teaching' (66). This view would be endorsed by McFarland and McFarlane (1989: 549) who state that: 'The ability of the nurse to identify and help correct a knowledge deficit is heavily influenced by her or his understanding of teaching and learning theories.' This would seem a reasonable assumption, but in the case of patient education how often are nurses' approaches to teaching influenced by their preferred theory of learning?

Conditioning learning theories

There are various ways of explaining how people learn and many theories have been proposed. They may be grouped into the broad categories of conditioning and cognitive theories. Those that relate to conditioning are based on associations between an organism receiving a stimulus and producing a response. The best known theory of this type is classical conditioning, described by Ivan Pavlov, a physiologist interested in digestion rather than education. He conducted laboratory-based experiments in which dogs salivated in response to food; this was an innate response, the dogs were not trained to do this. Under experimental conditions, Pavlov found that if he rang a bell before the dogs received the food he could train them to salivate when they heard the bell even in the absence of food. This was then known as a conditioned response. Lovell (1980) points out that while classical conditioning is a simple type of learning it plays an important role in the acquisition of emotions. Thus if a learning experience is associated with an unpleasant emotion, such as fear or anxiety, future behaviour may be influenced by the acquired emotion even though the emotion was not part of the intended learning experience. For example, if a woman attending an outpatient clinic for review of treatment of her angina was praised for losing some weight since her last appointment, she might develop a more positive association with attending the clinic, even though fostering her feelings about clinic attendance was not the primary goal. So while classical conditioning may not be of direct use in a health care setting it may have an indirect effect of either a positive or negative nature.

Leading on from this is the form of learning most often associated with the work of B.F. Skinner, in which training could be extended to get an animal to operate a lever in order to receive a reward, usually of food. This is a behavioural form of learning, known as operant conditioning. It can be used in a health care setting because behaviour could be modified through the provision of positive or negative reinforcement. Positive reinforcement involves giving a reward following a particular response. As a result, the response which has been rewarded will tend to increase in frequency. Perhaps the most frequently used form of positive reinforcement is verbal praise. Achieving one's own goals can also act as a form of positive reinforcement. By contrast, negative reinforcement involves the removal of some unpleasant stimulus following the occurrence of a desired response. For example, the reduction in anxiety which takes place when one leaves a frightening situation leads to an increased tendency to escape from or avoid such situations in the future, as in the case of the dental phobic who experiences a reduction in anxiety and pain on leaving the dentist's surgery. Thus, both positive and negative reinforcement increase the likelihood of a behaviour occurring. A third type of behavioural learning – punishment – involves either administering noxious stimuli or withdrawing a pleasant one. The effect of punishment is to decrease the likelihood of a behaviour occurring, and punishment is used (often ineffectively) in a myriad of mundane human situations, such as slapping or scolding a child for misbehaviour or withdrawing attention from elements of another's conversation (for example by looking away) which we are not interested in.

In a health care setting, people who have anorexia nervosa can be treated using operant conditioning approaches, where a rapid increase in weight is thought to be necessary. Increasing weight may be rewarded with treats or by reinstating previously withheld privileges such as listening to music (positive reinforcement). Negative reinforcement may also be offered, for example by allowing the patient to leave the (disliked) room in which she is nursed in return for weight gain. Third, weight loss could lead to some form of punishment, through the withdrawal of rewards which have previously been earned. It is proposed that by reinforcing the desired behaviour individuals will learn how to modify their behaviour in order to receive desired rewards. Although this form of treatment approach is rarely used today, it does illustrate how these three forms of operant conditioning can be combined in the clinical setting. A more current example involves the treatment of phobias and obsessions, both debilitating complaints to whose treatment both operant and classical conditioning have made the single most important contribution (Marks, 1977). In education, the actions of teachers who verbally praise desired responses from pupils represent almost universal instances of informal behavioural teaching/learning strategies.

Another form of operant conditioning is that of trial and error learning. One of the key investigators in this field was E.L. Thorndike who experimented with cats to find out how they would learn to find their food. By putting a hungry cat in a maze or a box the cat could eventually find how to reach its meal. Whilst it found its food initially by chance, through repeated trials the animal eventually learnt how the food was retrieved. One of the important outcomes of his work was the Law of Effect, which emphasises the importance of some sort of reward in acknowledgement of learning which has occurred (Lovell, 1980). Much of human learning is achieved through a trial and error approach in which a goal is achieved and this acts as a reward. However, in a health care setting trial and error may not be appropriate and indeed may be very dangerous. In some cases it would not be possible to risk any errors and in other situations there may be only one experience, for example, going to theatre, and therefore the patient cannot learn through trial and error. The fundamental additional contribution made by Skinner to this formulation of learning was the systematic application of rewards and punishments otherwise found through trial and error. Patient education generally aims to reduce the trial and error situation and hasten the formal learning component, except in situations where the process of growth in knowledge and awareness through the activities of trial and error is the desired outcome. In such situations, even trial and error is a goal-directed activity.

Both classical conditioning and operant learning are forms of associative learning in which the animal in an experimental situation learns to associate either a stimulus or an action with a reward. Arguably, this is a rather mechanistic approach to learning which excludes many attributes possessed by humans such as emotions and beliefs. It is also worth noting that often in health care any reward, in terms of health gain, may not be very obvious for a very long period of time. Indeed, the learning may only preserve the status quo. For example life style modification may reduce risk of heart problems or stopping smoking may reduce risk of respiratory problems. However, if people do not have such problems they may not perceive reducing 'risk' as a reward in itself. As a result, there may be no obvious natural reward in the short term, although people can reward themselves. For example, they may decide to allow themselves a treat if they do not smoke a cigarette for a week. Equally, the approval of some respected person may provide sufficient reinforcement to sustain valuable health behaviours in the absence of immediate rewards directly related to health gain.

Cognitive learning theories

To account for more complex forms of learning there are theories known as 'cognitive learning theories'. According to Ogier (1989: 117) 'Cognition is a term given to the mental processes such as thinking, problem-solving, remembering and perceiving.' This form of learning is often associated with the Gestalt approach to learning in which it is claimed that a reductionist approach to learning is not adequate and that the 'whole person's' experiences must be taken into account. Thus concepts such as perception and insight are important. Lovell (1980) explains the approach using the example of a cartoon:

> The Gestalt psychologists would have argued that no cartoon can be understood by analysing the individual strokes that make it up. The whole is greater than the sum of its parts. That extra element of meaningfulness that comes when we recognise five pencil strokes as the face of a well-known politician, for example, results from the four laws of perception.
>
> (43)

Gestalt learning theory is a form of cognitive theory. It is important in more complex situations and accounts for the way people learn from one situation and can then apply principles to another new situation and in this way can be said to have acquired problem solving skills. This approach to learning also helps to account for insight in which a person will suddenly see a solution or grasp a principle. Although not consciously developed at the time, insight is based on prior learning and knowledge, which is then brought into play in an entirely new situation. A well-known illustration of this is through the work of Kurt Kofka and W. Kohler, who put a chimpanzee in a cage with some boxes and a bunch of bananas which were suspended out of reach. After a while, the chimpanzee was seen to pile the boxes on top of each other, then climb up to them to reach the bananas. This was not the result of trial and error learning, rather, the authors suggested, the chimpanzee suddenly realised how he could solve the problem.

Another theory of learning from the cognitive camp is that of assimilation theory developed by David Ausubel in the 1950s and refined and developed by colleagues during the following twenty years (Ausubel *et al.*, 1978). It is termed assimilation theory to emphasise the importance of the 'interactive role that existing cognitive structures play in the process of new learning' (v). Although their theory of learning has been explicitly developed to explain school learning, some of their comments and principles appear to be applicable to teaching patients. They suggest that there are two main dimensions of classroom learning:

rote → meaningful learning
reception → discovery learning

Rote learning concerns where the learner acquires a set of information which is not particularly meaningful at the time and is not readily integrated into their existing stock of knowledge, for example learning multiplication tables. In contrast, meaningful learning is the acquisition of new material which can be readily integrated into existing cognitive material and abilities. Thus before teachers set out to deliver new material they should first ascertain what the individual already knows and then strive to give the new material in an organised way so that it can be integrated into his/her existing stock of knowledge. The importance of integrating new material on to old is emphasised in the introductory quotation, prior to the preface to the book: 'If I had to reduce all of educational psychology to just one principle, I would say this: The most important single factor influencing learning is what the learner already knows. Ascertain this and teach him accordingly' (Ausubel *et al.*, 1978).

Reception learning concerns the provision of new subject-matter in the 'final form'. Thus steps are taken to deliver the information in a format which learners can readily integrate into their stock of existing knowledge. It can be recalled later, or can be used as a foundation for further learning tasks. In contrast, in discovery learning the learner must find out for himself that which he is to learn. Discovery learning may be a more creative way to learn in which trial and error and problem solving are used. The authors argue that, on the whole, students learn by meaningful reception learning, that is, where the new material is explicitly designed to be integrated into existing knowledge and the presentation of the material is delivered in a way which facilitates this process. They do suggest, though, that in young children rote and discovery learning may be used more frequently.

Ausubel and colleagues establish that these are the principles underlying assimilation theory and throughout their book examine and challenge these ideas. While this theory has clearly been designed to explain classroom-based learning, the principle that people will learn most readily if steps are taken to establish what they already know and then teaching is organised in a way that new subject-matter is integrated into existing knowledge, also seems applicable to the needs of patients. There are differences, however, in the two situations. For example, Ausubel *et al.* state that in school learning the knowledge gained is often an end in itself, while in patient care information gain is rarely an end in itself; rather it is a means to another goal. In school learning the burden of the teaching responsibility belongs to teachers, to a greater degree than might be expected in a health care setting in which adults are encouraged to be active participants in the learning process. It can still be argued, however, that health care professionals are responsible for providing suitable educational opportunities for patients even when discovery learning rather than reception learning may be the goal.

The purpose of their book is to produce a psychological rationale for people who are aiming to increase the efficacy of their teaching, and this is surely both a laudable goal and highly relevant to the situation faced by health professionals. So, although some of the ideas in the assimilation theory may not be directly transferable to a health care situation, teachers are facing a parallel dilemma to that faced by nurses, who are grappling with the need to have a sound rationale for practice despite a lack of tried and tested theory to serve as a basis for practice. In the absence of suitable theory upon which to base teaching, teachers have to choose between: 'traditional prescriptions available in the educational folklore and on the precepts and examples of their own teachers and older colleagues. Or they can attempt to discover effective techniques of teaching through trial and error' (Ausubel *et al.*, 1978: 6). Neither of these approaches is supported in teaching and similarly neither are acceptable in nursing.

Gagne (1965), a cognitive theorist, argues that learning is a complex activity and that there are eight types of learning which form a hierarchy, progressing from relatively simple to difficult, as is shown in Figure 3.1. Signal and stimulus response learning are the lowest forms in this hierarchy whilst problem solving is at the top of the hierarchy. Lovell (1980) suggests that the hierarchy is useful in that it helps us to appreciate that there may be a natural progression from one stage to the next.

Thus, depending on what a person is supposed to learn, different learning theories may be most suitable and can then influence selection of a teaching strategy. For example, if a person is to take a tablet each morning a stimulus-response approach may be most suitable. The person would be asked to associate the new activity of taking their medication with an existing routine action so that the habitual action would remind them to undertake the new action. This activity should then be rewarded; this may be praise or some form of comfort they may not otherwise have. Receiving a reward would need to be continued until such time as the action became self-sustaining. Thus according to conditioned learning theorists, when teaching a person they must provide a stimulus to do the action and a reward after the action. In contrast, cognitive theorists must arrange new material in a way that the learners will make patterns and associations with it derived from earlier learning. Provision of new information must therefore be carefully planned to build upon existing knowledge and associations. New material must be grouped and presented in a way that will facilitate the learner grasping the information or situation and interpreting it in the light of previous experiences.

The limitations of conditioning and cognitive learning theories

It was stated at the start of this section that theory is not the same as science and that theory must be proved. Whilst the above theories seem plausible it is also important to consider their shortcomings. In particular they may be criticised for being largely developed in laboratory rather than empirical, real-life, situations. Second, many were developed using animals or by focusing on the needs of children. Third, general educational principles may not readily transfer to the health care situation. As Luker and Caress (1989: 712) have pointed out: 'the applicability of mainstream educational principles to the teaching of patients who, by definition, are sick is questionable, and in many cases unworkable'.

The transference of these learning theories to health care settings should not be taken for granted but should be tested. There are other controversies and criticisms surrounding human learning. For example, Rogers (1969) has a completely different approach, which Ogier (1989: 121) has categorised as a form of humanistic theory: 'Humanistic theories are concerned with human growth, individual fulfilment and self-actualisation. The emphasis of the theories is on teacher–student relationship and the learning climate.'

Type 1	Signal learning	The individual learns to make a general, diffuse response to a signal. This is the classical conditioned response of Pavlov.
Type 2	Stimulus response learning	The learner acquires a precise response to a particular stimulus. What is learned is a connection (Thorndike) or a discriminating operant response (Skinner).
Type 3	Chaining	What is acquired is a chain of two or more stimulus-response connections.
Type 4	Verbal association	The learning of chains that are verbal. Basically, the conditions resemble those for other chains. However, the presence of language in human beings makes this a special type because internal links may be selected from the individual's previously learned repertoire of language.
Type 5	Multiple discrimination	The individual learns to make n different identifying responses to as many different stimuli, which may resemble each other in physical appearance to a greater or lesser degree.
Type 6	Concept learning	The learner acquires the capability of making a common response to a class of stimuli that may differ from each other widely in physical appearance. He is able to make a response that identifies an entire class of objects or events.
Type 7	Principle learning	In simplest terms, a principle is a chain of two or more concepts. It

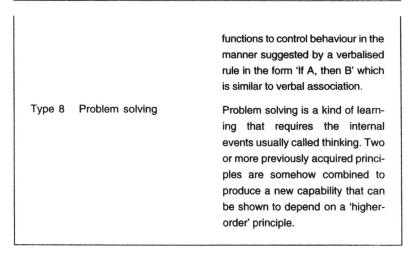

		functions to control behaviour in the manner suggested by a verbalised rule in the form 'If A, then B' which is similar to verbal association.
Type 8	Problem solving	Problem solving is a kind of learning that requires the internal events usually called thinking. Two or more previously acquired principles are somehow combined to produce a new capability that can be shown to depend on a 'higher-order' principle.

Figure 3.1 Gagne's proposed types of learning
Source: Gagne, 1965: 58–59.

Rogers suggests that teaching can be interpreted as simply instructing and as such is not a complex activity. However, he argues that, as the environment changes rapidly, instruction has a very limited use. Instead he believes that the role of teachers is to enable adults to learn for themselves. They can then continue learning and adapt as their circumstances change. This then affects the teaching process because, he argues, teachers must work from a basis of genuineness, trust and respect and be able to empathise and understand the learner through good listening skills. The guidelines which Rogers therefore suggests are to do with:

- creating an appropriate climate to facilitate learners
- making learning resources readily available to the learners
- allowing the teacher to be used as a resource by learners
- the teacher as facilitator becoming one of the group, learning alongside the learners.

The work of Maslow (1970) who proposed that education should aim to help individuals to make the most of themselves would also belong in this category (Ogier, 1989).

Nurses reading these outlines of theories may be able to identify patients from their own experience who may have benefited from one of the approaches above but not from another. Thus it is likely that no single theory of learning or teaching would suffice for all aspects of patient education.

Adult education – the concept of andragogy

As the focus of this book is adults rather than children the work of Knowles (1980) regarding adult learners seems relevant. The work of Malcolm Knowles, from the discipline of education, attempts to explain how adults learn. Knowles uses the word *andragogy* to describe 'the art and science of helping adults learn' as opposed to *pedagogy* which concerns the teaching of children. Overall, the development of theories of adult learning is still in its infancy (Merriam, 1987) and there is no consensus of opinion regarding the most useful theory. It is argued by Pratt (1988) that Knowles' work is not sufficiently developed to be a theory, while Merriam (1988) states that the assumptions are not all unique to adults and therefore cannot be called a theory of adult learning specifically. However, the main assumptions proposed by Knowles regarding adult learners seem plausible, applicable and potentially useful to the situation of patient education. They are as follows:

1   *The need to know.* Adults need to know why they need to learn something before they will learn it.
2   *The learner's self-concept.* Adults have a self-concept that they are responsible for their own decisions, for their own lives. They need to be seen by others as self-directing. They tend to resist others imposing their will upon them.
3   *The role of the learner's experience.* Adults arrive in an educational setting with past experiences which will have a bearing upon the immediate situation.
4   *Readiness to learn.* Adults become ready to learn those things they need to know and be able to do in order to cope effectively with their real-life situations.
5   *Orientation to learning.* In contrast to younger peoples' subject-centred orientation to learning, adults are life-centred. Adults are motivated to learn something if they believe it will help them undertake real-life situations.

1 The need to know	The reason for the education must be explained so that individuals can understand why it is thought to be relevant to their needs.
2 The learner's self-concept	When planning to teach adults new information take into account their self-perception. For example, whether they wish to be autonomous decision makers or passive participants in their care, this is likely to influence the volume of information they would want to receive. A patient's self-concept may also influence choice teaching intervention, e.g. whether they wish to direct the learning by asking questions, whether they wish to be left booklets or whether they want teaching paced by health professionals.
3 The role of the learner's experience	When assessing the person check prior knowledge, skills, views, on the subject and its source. Take former learning into account and build on it. This will help foster partnerships because the individual will realise that you are not assuming they are ignorant of all information, indeed the patient may end up teaching the nurse. Attitudes and beliefs will also be influenced by prior experience and must be taken into account.
4 Readiness to learn	Aim to pace education to match readiness to learn. Appraise patient's current situation e.g. A&E, pre-op, prior to discharge, at home and try to arrange education to suit. Avoid overwhelming patients with information; small and often may be more effective than a single but lengthy teaching session. If patients indicate verbally or non-verbally that they are unable or unwilling to learn at a particular time consider how patient education needs could be met at another time. It is inappropriate to plan to teach people who are not ready to learn.
5 Orientation to learning	Aim to link education to patients' own goals and aspirations to other aspects of their life. Discuss how proposed education could help them to achieve professional, social or personal goals. Aim to place new information and skills in the broader context of a person's life rather than simply related to a health issue as though it is independent of other aspects of their life.
6 Motivation	Notice verbal and non-verbal cues to help gauge how well motivated a person may be and plan education accordingly. If person is not well motivated try to discover underlying reasons. These are usually internal factors. Seek motivating factors and link education to include these.

Figure 3.2 Knowles' assumptions about adult learning

Source: From *The Adult Learner: A Neglected Species*, 4th edn by Malcolm Knowles. Copyright © 1990 by Gulf Publishing Company. Used with permission. All rights reserved.

6 *Motivation.* While adults are responsive to some external motivators, such as a better job, the most potent motivators are internal pressures, e.g. increased job satisfaction, quality of life.

(Knowles, 1990: 57–63)

By taking each of these assumptions about the adult learner into account, the principles underlying teaching adults are also apparent and appear to be transferable to the context of teaching adult patients.

Other theories of adult learning have been developed, but as Merriam (1987) points out, few have been tested and none are supported by a body of research evidence. However, the work of Knowles has been widely applied, and the assumptions listed above can offer useful points which can be applied to patient education. Only by using such work and evaluating it in practice will its value be confirmed or refuted. Perhaps different theory will prove to be useful in different settings. As Szasz and Hollender (1956) suggested, in critical care an activity passivity model may be most expedient when patients limited by physiological instability may be unable to participate in any form of teaching programme. But they may be able to absorb information passively to be aware of what is to happen to them. This approach progresses to the guidance co-operation model for people in non-emergency situations and then to that of mutual participation for people in chronic illness situations. Clearly, critically ill patients may not be able to be self-directing in their learning as is suggested by Knowles (1990). However, it must be remembered that his work was not originally developed for a patient/health care setting so its application to such a setting must be carefully evaluated.

As Pratt (1988) points out: 'What is important however, is the element of informed intentional choice: self-directed learners have to decide, first, if they value having control and second, if they will do anything to either establish or relinquish that control' (170). Thus Knowles' second assumption that adults are self-directing is still important as it allows them the right to have control over their learning. However, through assessment, the nurse can determine whether in some situations patients may relinquish this right to self-direction. Clearly, care and sensitivity will be needed to assure that the patient is not mistakenly thought to either wish or need to relinquish this right. In this sense, Knowles' second assumption may still serve as a useful guide to how nurses should perceive adult learners.

While the work of Knowles may not be accepted as a theory, it can offer nurses an insight into how educational interventions may be organised to enhance adults' learning, as has been suggested in Figure 3.2. If the principles are robust then they should be applicable to health as well as educational settings. Only by using them and testing them will the body of evidence to support or refute the work of Knowles in health care settings be developed.

Learning theories and teaching theories

To illustrate how the concept of learning precedes the approach to teaching, Anderson's (1986) 'bucket theory' will be mentioned. In the bucket theory, knowledge, which may comprise such elements as information, skills and attitudes, is within the educator and outside the patient.

> The purpose of education is to get these elements inside the patient; if the right combination of these elements can be internalised by patients, they will comply with the prescribed regimen. In this view of education the educator functions as a full bucket trying to pour knowledge into the patient, i.e. the empty bucket.
>
> (85)

If this theory is subscribed to then the educator will plan teaching sessions in a teacher-centred rather than a learner-centred way. Little attention may be given to the patients' own perspectives about what they most want to learn, or about prior learning and experience as it will be assumed that the teacher has all the facts. The teacher will then concentrate on how best to transfer his or her own knowledge to the patient. Although the bucket theory is something of a parody it helps to illustrate the link between learning theory and subsequent educational intervention. Alternatively, there are others who support a more patient-centred approach to learning by building upon existing knowledge. Coles (1989) argues that if a person has a great deal of new information to master then a lego-building approach, using small units of information which link into each other, is more likely to be successful than a bucket-filling approach. By reflecting back on the learning theories mentioned above, the basis for his argument can be supported by the principles of cognitive theory.

Types of learning

It is widely accepted that there are three types of learning. These are:

- *Cognitive learning* – which is about acquiring information and thought processes;
- *Affective learning* – which is about emotions and beliefs. These factors will have an influence on whether information is learnt or put into practice; thus affective learning may alter an individual's attitudes towards their health problem or reinforce a positive belief;
- *Psychomotor skill learning* – which involves performing tasks such as giving an injection, or applying a dressing.

(Kiger, 1995)

All these types of learning may be required in a patient education setting and all will require a different teaching approach. The types of learning to be achieved will be identified when assessing the patient. The information covered in Chapters 4 and 5 relates most closely to cognitive forms of learning and Chapters 6 and 7 to affective learning, although they are not arranged to deal with these topics specifically. Relatively little research-based information is available about teaching psychomotor skills to patients and this represents an area in urgent need of development.

Conclusion

In this chapter a résumé of broad categories of learning theories has been presented and related to patient education. The way in which a nurse believes a patient will learn should influence the teaching strategies used. While the theories of education presented in this chapter may be used to inform practice they are largely untested in the context of patient care, and therefore should be used and tested with a view to increasing the body of knowledge relating to patient education. Kappeli (1993) urges us to exploit knowledge developed by other disciplines and in this sense testing whether learning theory is useful in nursing practice is a valuable endeavour. However, it must also be noted that nursing is a practice activity and that, therefore, any theories used must be easily applicable in practice. As Kappeli, drawing from the work of Audrey Miller, has noted, the theory practice gap is an enduring problem because the practice settings in which nurses work are so different to the educational and research institutions in which theory tends to be discussed. Thus in practice: 'nursing is what nurses do while, in theory, nursing is what nurses ought to do regardless of any context, spatial or time conditions' (Kappeli, 1993: 207).

Theory which is not valuable and applicable in practice is not useful in nursing. The point of discussing education theory is not to suggest that it can be automatically transferred to nursing situations, but that nurses need to consider the theoretical basis for practice and modify existing theories to suit, or to develop new ideas from practice.

KEY POINTS FROM CHAPTER THREE

1   *Research, theory and practice should be interdependent* in patient education. Practice which does not have a theoretical basis to guide it, or research evidence to support it will be less defensible and have a less obvious rationale than if all elements are in play.

2   *Behavioural, cognitive and humanistic approaches to learning provide different perspectives* which may be useful in different patient education situations.

3   *Theories of adult learning* have been developed in the disciplines of education and psychology and may be applicable to patient education settings. There are no theories specifically developed to explain and predict patient education processes.

4   *Nurses should be involved in theory development* relating to patient education to help strengthen the knowledge base of nursing.

5   *The concept of andragogy* developed by Malcolm Knowles appears to be particularly applicable to patient education situations and warrants application and testing.

Chapter 4

Teaching strategies I: assessment and planning

Introduction

Although it is generally agreed that teaching is an important activity, it is reported that such teaching is often done on an unplanned and unstructured basis, with little attempt at evaluation of impact upon the patient. Thus it can be difficult to defend patient teaching as an essential part of care because we are frequently unable to prove its value in tangible terms. The only way to improve this situation is to learn from people who have conducted rigorous research into patient education and have reported the results. In this chapter and the next, a wide range of literature will be consulted to identify points for good practice, drawn from a variety of sources and will be presented as a guide to developing effective but realistic patient teaching. The focus will primarily be on patient education in the acute sector – mainly hospitals and outpatient clinics. However, many of the points will also be applicable to primary care settings. As the range of settings in which patient education may occur is so vast it is difficult to suggest universally applicable guidelines. Clearly, the needs of patients and therefore the patient education required will be variable according to the nature of their illness, the context in which their care is to be provided and individuals' own perceptions and situations.

These two chapters provide a general overview relating to teaching adults with physical health problems. The specific needs of children, people with learning disabilities or mental health problems are not the focus of this book. The focus of this chapter is particularly on aspects of patient education relating to assessment and planning. It is intended that some of the points raised will link to the previous chapter on learning theories and throughout this chapter research-based findings will be presented. By so doing the aim is to help link theory and research together to indicate points for good practice. The chapter will also be closely linked to Chapter 5, which suggests how the activities of assessment and planning can be translated into actual teaching and its evaluation.

The influence of the current health care climate upon patient education will be considered first, to recognise the context in which patient education must often occur. Then, to provide a structure for the process of patient teaching, relevant material will be considered under the following sections: assessment, identification of needs/ nursing diagnosis, goals, intervention and evaluation. The process of teaching is similar to that of the nursing process and in both the assessment and evaluation stages often occurs continually rather than in a linear fashion. An example of the standard to be aimed for will be illustrated by including patient education standards developed to enhance the education of patients with arthritis and musculoskeletal problems. These are an outstanding set of standards and are included to indicate the degree of rigour and thought that needs to be applied to patient education in practice.

Current health care climate and patient education

In the current health care climate patients are in hospital for as short a stay as is possible. Thus while they are inpatients they may be too ill to receive patient education. They are discharged speedily, often before they are recovered, and must rapidly learn to care for themselves. In addition, there are fewer qualified nurses in the clinical areas due to skill-mix policies and resources for patient education are constrained. As patients now stay in hospital for less time than they used to there is limited time in which patient education can occur. Furthermore, acutely ill patients do not have the physiological stability, energy or concentration to learn about care during much of their time in hospital (Bubela *et al.*, 1990).

Ruzicki (1989) pointed out that the challenge of meeting the educational needs of very ill patients who are in hospital for only a short time is enormous. Almost ten years later the situation is, if anything, even more acute. Nurses are working with increasingly ill patients. Due to skill-mix policies it is likely that, once stable, patients will be cared for by assistants whilst qualified nurses remain with the most ill and unstable individuals. For physiologically unstable individuals patient education must take a lower priority. To work within such constraints Ruzicki (1989: 629) suggests that 'ideal is out, realistic is in' and that nurses must 'get real' if patient education is to occur at all.

> Nurses must revise their expectations of themselves and adopt an abbreviated, efficient and expeditious form of patient educa-tion – likely different from what they learned in school.
>
> (Ruzicki, 1989: 629)

Despite her call for an abbreviated form of education, Ruzicki still recommends that nurses must involve both a process and a struc-ture in their patient education and in particular she recommends thorough assessment of need. Only by collecting accurate assess-ment data can realistic priorities be identified. In the long run this may save time as it may prevent nurses from inappropriate teaching which is a waste of time.

Thus while accepting that patient education must be compressed into a shorter space of time than is ideal, the need for thorough, planned, good quality teaching remains. This chapter will aim to identify teaching initiatives which can be supported by research and yet are applicable to the constraints under which most nurses work.

Assessment of patients' needs for education

It is advocated in this book that a thorough assessment of patients' needs must be undertaken prior to planning any teaching interven-tions. Clearly the assessment format must be compatible with the totality of nurses' work. It would not be feasible for rating scales to be applied to every item raised below. In some situations however, assessment instruments may be applicable. By discussing the need for assessment specifically, the intention is to emphasise the importance of this aspect of care. The general principle should be that some form of assessment is always undertaken prior to initi-ating an educational intervention with patients, since education may be considered a form of 'treatment' in just the same way as any other part of a nurse's clinical work. The formality and extent of the assessment will, of course, vary according to the situation, and the existence of evidence to guide the assessment process.

What do patients want to know?

The importance of a thorough assessment is of vital importance if appropriate patient education is to be arranged. For example, after a meta-analysis based on 68 studies to examine the effect of pre-operative instruction on post-operative outcomes Hathaway (1986) concluded that,

> a preoperative instruction based on individual learners' needs would, by addressing the specific needs of the individual have a greater positive effect on postoperative outcomes. In addition, by focusing on each patient's specific needs, greater consistency in the effectiveness of preoperative instruction could be expected.
>
> (274)

Thus we cannot assume that all patients require the same education even though they may be admitted for a similar form of medical intervention. In addition, assessment enables needs to be prioritised and care to be focused. This may save time and money in the long run as patients will not be subjected to teaching they don't want, on topics they are not interested in, at a time they are not ready to learn. The chances of effective and efficient care being delivered are increased if patients' needs are thoroughly understood by those providing the care. Assessment to find out vital information is the first step in patient education. Items of information which patients are likely to be interested in are illustrated below in Figure 4.1.

Although none of these issues can be assumed or taken for granted, how often have nurses presumed to tell patients what they think they need to know? Dalayon (1994) investigated perceived needs of surgical patients in Kuwait and found patients had different priorities to the nurses. Patients' most highly rated information needs were:

- how to care for their wound at home
- how to turn in bed
- how to get in and out of bed
- explanations about their measurements of their vital signs, and
- general information about their wound

- what an individual needs to know and be able to do
- what type of individual information is needed prior to discharge
- whether the person is ready to learn
- previous learning to identify factors which will influence learning (such as extent of desire for independence, past experiences, social expectations)
- what must they do when they get home
- what skills must they have at home
- what must they know to be safe
- what must they have until supplementary education can be offered
- how do they learn
- whether they wish to be active decision makers
- are there any factors which will influence learning such as physical disabilities or intellectual capacity
- cultural influences.

Figure 4.1   What patients may want to know

In contrast, nurses ranked the following items as most important:

- the need for early ambulation, deep breathing and coughing exercises
- pre-operative procedures
- fasting and changes in food intake
- care of the wound after discharge

The patients' list would support the assumption of Knowles (1990) [discussed in Chapter 3], as it illustrates that patients want to know about what they have to do. They may need this information before they feel ready to absorb any other.

Dalayon's results suggest that nurses' teaching is done with a view to preventing post-operative complications, which is, of course, important. Unfortunately, the patients are focusing on a rather different set of needs. This study is illustrative of the need to prepare teaching to ensure that both nurses' and patients' priorities are met. As the work of Anderson (1986) (discussed in Chapter 3) suggests, education needs to be patient-centred rather than educator-centred if it is to be most successful. Patients' views must be taken into account if patient satisfaction is to be achieved. Other work has also identified that patients and nurses may perceive learning needs quite differently (Herbert, 1997; Ojanlatva *et al.*, 1997; Anderson *et al.*, 1993; Lauer *et al.*, 1982).

Furthermore, learning needs change as patients' situations alter; thus assessment must be ongoing. Bostrom *et al.* (1994) investigated the perceived learning needs of patients in hospital and those who were recently discharged. They used the Patient Learning Need Scale developed by Bubela *et al.* (1990) and 76 inpatients and 89 recently discharged individuals participated. Information about medications, treatment and complications, and enhanced quality of life (symptom management) had top priority with people in hospital. Information on activities of living, community follow-up, skin care and feelings about their condition was not ranked so highly. Recently discharged patients rated the types of information in a similar order but rated the importance of the categories of information more highly. Thus need for information increases rather than decreases among the recently discharged.

The patients wanted practically applicable information rather than physiology and anatomy relating to their condition. Patients do not appear to want the theoretical underpinnings of their condition. Clark (1994) reviewed research-based literature concerning educational interventions for patients with asthma. Teaching relating to self-management instructions was considered more successful than general education about the disease process. This perceived need for information that is practically applicable is in keeping with Knowles' (1990) assumptions as previously discussed (see Chapter 3).

Bubela *et al.* (1990) assessed factors influencing patients' perceived learning needs on discharge from hospital. They developed and used the Patient Learning Need Scale, comprising 50 self-administered items, and patients were asked to rate each item according to how important they felt it would be for them to know about at home. Informational needs were not found to be affected by age, marital status, home situation or health but were affected by 'gender, level of education, number of medications, type of illness experience and perceptions about the effect that their illness would have on their life' (25). They found that greater informational needs may be seen at discharge in patients who are female; of low and middle level education; have been diagnosed with cancer; and have extensive medication regimens (Bubela *et al.*, 1990: 27).

They stressed the importance of being able to prioritise information and thus not waste time. They recommended that studies are conducted with specific patient populations to allow greater understanding of their pre- and post-discharge information requirements. The needs of several specific patient populations have been investigated but not both before and after discharge. For example, Goodman (1997) investigated patients' perceptions of their learning needs during the first six weeks after discharge from hospital following cardiac surgery. Through her experience in cardiac care and from the literature she was aware that there was a definite need for educational follow-up. Only ten patients were involved in the study but these people were interviewed at their six-week post-operative outpatient appointment and also completed a diary to document their educational needs. The areas which the patients identified as important were:

- pain relief
- sleep promotion
- limitations to activity (e.g. difficulty with dressing, brushing hair)
- lack of information (e.g. about TED stockings, aperients, driving)
- exercising
- dietary needs
- medication
- negative psychological states (e.g. feeling low, apathetic, weepy, depressed)
- positive psychological states (e.g. feeling of euphoria at being able to resume old activities such as going out for a walk without getting angina)
- community support links
- owning responsibility for care.

Recommendations were drawn up as a result of this investigation to have these issues addressed in future discharge planning and education. This work is interesting, but its applicability is somewhat constrained by the small sample size. The work of Mistiaen et al. (1997) and Jaarsma et al. (1995) also supports the need for ongoing patient education post-discharge and emphasises the need to re-assess patients at different stages of their treatment and recovery as their educational requirements will change.

Some patients have been found to be particularly disadvantaged when considering their informational needs. For example, the Audit Commission (1993: 10) report that the following patients experienced the greatest difficulties in receiving general information:

- disabled patients using wheelchairs
- patients with visual impairments
- patients who are deaf or who are hard of hearing
- patients who do not speak English
- elderly patients who are mentally ill
- patients with learning disabilities

This list suggests that when nurses are planning patient education for particular client groups these particular needs must be catered for. Nurses need to find out what in particular prevents those in wheelchairs getting access to necessary information. Is it structural? Does the design of outpatients' clinics or hospital facilities, for example, prevent them from reaching sources of information? Could patients with visual impairments have access to tape-recorded information, or could leaflets be transcribed on to braille sheets for the blind? Patients who are deaf need access to videos, written material or equivalent information in visually explicit ways. Similarly for the other points listed, ways must be sought to help overcome barriers posed for those with physical or mental problems. It should always be remembered that nurses could engage the help of charitable organisations to help in this form of work, for example, by working with the Royal Institute for the Blind to access additional advice and resources to help their particular client group. While this creates extra work for nurses, it would be indefensible simply to disregard the needs of these people when we have explicit information to indicate that they are currently disadvantaged in the arena of patient education.

In addition to the points made above it must be remembered that the current health care climate, as previously discussed, does not lend itself to enhancing learning opportunities. As patients tend to spend less time with health professionals, the need to prioritise learning needs increases. As Ruzicki (1989) has commented, patients may be able to absorb very little information in hospital so nurses must carefully consider what is essential whilst patients are unstable or are not able to learn. However, the finding that informational needs are increased rather than decreased around the time for discharge helps stress the need for follow-up care. Nurses must therefore assess hospital needs for education and project ahead to anticipate learning needs for discharged patients. Strategies for long-term behavioural change must be planned for and integrated into care but it must be accepted that they must be given later rather than in the acute situation.

Whilst patients should not be completely stereotyped according to their medical condition it is reasonable to assume that they will have some learning needs in common. The work of Graydon *et al.* (1997) on the needs of those with breast cancer; Hagenhoff *et al.* (1994) with respect to the needs of people with congestive cardiac failure; Jaarsma *et al.* (1995) regarding patients post-myocardial infarction or coronary by-pass grafting; or Hill (1997) relating to patients with rheumatoid arthritis, has begun to establish potential needs in the respective client groups. Where rigorous research is available it offers a golden opportunity to learn from and build upon the work of others. Such reports can be examined to see if they can be applied by nurses at local levels.

Readiness to learn

Pohl (1965) defined '"readiness" to learn as the person's physical and mental ability to learn viewed in terms of his neuro-muscular developments' and saw these two concepts of ability as being 'the patient wanting to learn – his motivation', and 'whether he is able to learn – his readiness'.

Therefore, in addition to assessing the type of information patients require, it is generally recognised that it is important to assess whether they are ready to learn. For example, fear is an important factor when assessing learning priorities because frightened individuals will not learn. If patients are still shocked after hearing their diagnosis they may not be able to retain any further information given to them (Beaver and Luker, 1997).

If patients are not ready to learn it is a waste of time and resources to go through an educational programme with them just so that it can be said to have been delivered. In contrast, if an individual's readiness to learn is taken into account and patient education offered when the patient is receptive to it, the intervention may be more effective and thus 'more cost-effective than randomly teaching at the convenience of health-care providers or in accordance with the policies of a hospital or other health care institution' (Vanetzian, 1997: 593).

Physical	Pain, fatigue, sensory deprivation
Psychological	Motivation, attitude, beliefs about illness, emotional response to illness, e.g. fear or shock
Intellectual	Literacy, ability to comprehend
Socioeconomic/cultural	Ethnicity, religious beliefs, health values, family roles/relationships, support structures, financial concerns, home environment.

Figure 4.2 Factors affecting readiness to learn

According to Ruzicki (1989: 631), several factors can be expected to have an effect upon educational readiness and they are illustrated in Figure 4.2. These factors are supported by the work of others (Redman, 1984; De Muth, 1989; Vanetzian, 1997). Patients' actual health condition may also influence readiness to learn and must be taken into account (Vanetzian, 1997). Nurses working in their particular clinical area and health care setting are best able to predict what factors are most likely to affect their own clients, for example, following a diagnosis of cancer or heart disease, and they can then refine these rather generic factors during individual assessments.

The hierarchy of needs proposed by Maslow (1970) also has a place in helping us to appreciate individuals' readiness to learn and learning needs. Maslow proposes that humans have the following hierarchy of needs:

1   Physiological and survival needs
2   Safety and security
3   Love, affection, belongingness
4   Esteem
5   Self-actualisation

The physical needs take priority over all others. Thus physiological needs must be met first. They include the need for food and water, warmth and shelter, without which we are likely to die. Safety needs include having protection from danger. Social needs include our desire to belong to a group and to be accepted by others; we need friends and companionship. Self-esteem concerns our need to feel we are productive and useful, which enables us to have a sense of being respected. Self-actualisation is the final layer of Maslow's hierarchy and relates to our desire of becoming all that we are capable of. It includes being creative (Messenger, 1992).

This hierarchy informs us that until basic needs for survival are met higher order needs are not considered. According to Maslow, as soon as one level of need is met another takes its place, but it is unlikely that a higher need would be met before a lower one was satisfied. Thus for patients who are critically ill, patient education is inappropriate. Similarly, education about basic safety and security is required before any other form of information is needed. This model was supported by the findings of Derdiarian (1986) with reference to informational needs of recently diagnosed cancer patients.

Luker and Caress (1989) also stress the importance of physiological needs in patient education and point out that biochemical changes experienced by sick individuals may greatly erode their ability to learn. For example, patients in end-stage renal failure may be considered by health professionals to be in serious need of education in order to understand renal dialysis, but cognitive ability may be severely reduced secondary to fluid and biochemical imbalance. Luker and Caress argue that the physiological influences upon learning have largely been overlooked in the literature on assessment of patients' learning needs and readiness to learn and that a decade later extensive literature searches suggest that situation is largely unchanged. They note that in our need to ensure that psychological needs are not overlooked we have created an imbalance in which physiological effects upon learning may easily be overlooked:

> in moving towards holism, nurses must remember that in many circumstances if the patient is not able to maintain his physical well-being, attention to the psychological will become redundant – since the patient will have ceased to be!
>
> (Luker and Caress, 1989: 714)

Patients' readiness to learn will influence the timing of their teaching. Tilley *et al.* (1987) report that patients are receptive to information about their illness immediately after admission, the type of information which they want at this time being that which has immediate and personal relevance. As a result of their study they recommend that:

The nurse's role during the early part of the patient's hospital-ization should be to provide the type of information patients desire in order to make sense of their illness experience at that time.

(299)

This would concur with the theoretical perspective advocated by Knowles (1990), as has already been discussed in Chapter 3.

It is often assumed that this process can only begin once indi-viduals have been admitted for care. However, several authors have reported that giving information prior to hospital admission or commencing treatment can be a successful strategy (Butow *et al.*, 1998; Scriven and Tucker, 1997; Theis and Johnson, 1995; Roach *et al.*, 1995; Tooth and McKenna, 1995; Mikulaninec, 1987). Theis and Johnson (1995) estimated the effects of pre-admission and post-admission teaching and found they were both influential. Thus nurses can be confident that pre-admission teaching is a valuable strategy: it is as effective as the more conventional post-admission teaching and may save time in acute settings for planned admis-sions. Thus in terms of readiness to learn, for people needing planned surgery the optimal time may be prior to admission, because once admitted people may have too much on their mind to absorb information presented to them. This strategy would also appear to help overcome the problem of severe time constraints upon teaching within a hospital setting. This may be an area for development for specialist nurses who may have more freedom and autonomy to organise teaching outside the conventional hospital inpatient period.

In order to assess readiness to learn, in the absence of anything more sophisticated, nurses can ask fundamental questions such as:

'Would you like me to tell you about how we prepare you for your operation?'
'Do you feel ready to learn about your leg ulcer today?'
'Are you in the mood to learn about changing your stoma bag now?'
'Can you tell me what concerns you most about your discharge home?'
'Do you wish to hear about the types of exercise we recom-mend you take when you go home?'
'Do you want to be consulted about all changes in your treat-ment regimen?'

By paying attention to patients' verbal and non-verbal responses it should be possible to gauge whether patients wish to learn. The important point is that nurses realise that such questions are important, that patients should have some say in the scheduling of their teaching and that it is unwise to force information upon patients who are not receptive to it. Such activity would be a waste of both the patient's and the nurse's time. Similarly, nurses must be observant of patients' behaviour. Patients who are in pain or preoccupied by other worries are unlikely to be receptive to fresh information. Balanced against this, there may be occasions when even patients who are indeed likely to be resistant to information need it in order to preserve their safety.

While the approach to assessment described in the previous paragraph may not be considered to be highly scientific, verbal and non-verbal communication skills are the essential starting point for most aspects of nursing care. Such skills, plus experience and insight, enable nurses to make clinical decisions for individual patients. There will never be a protocol for each nursing action; professional judgement will always play some part in nursing care.

Involvement in care

In the assessment nurses should attempt to gauge the extent to which patients wish to be involved in making decisions about their treatment. In Chapter 1, patient involvement in decision making was discussed and from previous work it seems that patient participation cannot be assumed. Therefore, individual preferences need to be understood as this will influence the focus of the educational intervention. Neufeld *et al.* (1993) describe how they assessed patients' opinions about participation using a series of five-option choice cards, ranging from a highly active role to a totally passive role in which the patient would elect that the doctor made all decisions about treatment. The approach was thought to work well when used with women with a diagnosis of breast or gynaecological cancer. These treatment choices were then taken into account when planning future teaching and care.

Types of learner

Several authors have reported that individuals may have different styles of learning (Kolb, 1976; Jarvis and Gibson, 1985; Honey and

Mumford, 1986). According to Honey and Mumford (1986) there are four main learning styles:

1   The activist learner who does best when actively involved in the process; they need the opportunity to 'have a go' whilst still being guided and protected.
2   The reflective learner who needs time to think back over the problem.
3   The theorist who needs to understand the theoretical basis of what they are learning rather than just an application of it.
4   The pragmatists who are said to learn best from an appropriate role model.

Alternatively Jarvis and Gibson (1985: 47) suggest the types of learning styles displayed in Figure 4.3.

These frameworks are included as examples, but they are not proven. Indeed it is important that they are empirically tested so that their impact on learning outcomes can be estimated. Most of us probably adopt different styles in different situations and may not be at the extremes of the continuum. Frameworks such as these

---

Concrete versus abstract: some learners like to start with a concrete situation such as experience, while others prefer to commence with an abstract, theoretical idea.

Converger versus diverger: the converger is best in situations where there is a single correct solution, whereas divergers are best in situations where they can generate ideas and broad perspectives.

Focusing and scanning: focusers examine problems as a totality whereas scanners select one aspect of the problem and assume it is the solution until further information disproves it.

Holistic versus serialistic: some learners see a phenomenon as a whole while others prefer to string together the parts.

Impulsivity versus reflectivity: some learners respond first and reflect later while others reflect first and respond later.

Figure 4.3 Learning styles suggested by Jarvis and Gibson

Source: From *The Teacher Practitioner in Nursing, Midwifery and Health Visiting* by P. Jarvis and S. Gibson (1985). Used with permission of Croom Helm.

are important when designing teaching strategies for students. Whether it will ever be possible to modify teaching interventions to suit patients' preferences in a health care setting is debatable. On one hand we barely have time to assess to this depth, and having done so it would imply that a range of teaching approaches was available and the nurse could select the one deemed most suitable at the time. This may not be feasible. On the other hand if we try to teach someone using an intervention which does not appeal to them the chance of the desired learning taking place decreases. It is only worth assessing learning styles, however, if teaching strategies can be modified accordingly. It appears that assessment of learning styles would be more appropriate in those with a chronic rather than an acute condition.

Conducting the assessment

The two main ways we can assess patients' needs for education are via an interview and through careful observation. Assessment through interview may occur on admission to hospital or on first contact with a patient but is then likely to be ongoing during any further contact there is with the patient. Assessment can be informal or formal and structured according to the health care setting in which it is conducted. Information can be gathered when involved with other care, such as helping a patient to get washed or dressed, or when changing a dressing. The type of data gathered may be influenced by the documentation used by nurses, for example, if a particular proforma is used, if any model of nursing is followed or whether individualised or standardised care plans are available.

Assessment is a continuous process; it can begin prior to admission for planned cases, then be ongoing during a hospital stay and continue when the patient returns to the community. For emergency admissions it will be undertaken whilst providing care for patients. If it is not possible to gain information from the patient it may be gained from family or next of kin.

Factors which can influence the conduct of an assessment may include age, language, literacy, prior knowledge, disease, mental state. What appears to be vital is that at the assessment stage patients are treated as individuals and each person's unique profile is taken into consideration (Tooth and McKenna, 1995).

On the part of the nurse the skills that may be required to conduct the assessment include:

- observation
- interviewing
- priority setting
- problem solving
- communication skills

(Marks-Maran *et al.*, 1988)

It is likely that all assessments will involve some interviewing and to do this well nurses must have good interpersonal skills and communication skills. The assessment interview is often the first meeting of the nurse and the patient and will influence all future interactions. Dickson *et al.* (1997) analyse the actual skills required in interpersonal communication and discuss in detail how the following skills can be enhanced:

- non-verbal communication
- reinforcement
- questioning
- reflecting
- starting and ending an interaction
- explanation

Each of these skills and techniques has been supported and explained using a wealth of literature. Similarly Newell (1994) discusses interviewing skills in great detail. Communication skills and the art of successful assessment are a subject in themselves and beyond the remit of this book. Fortunately, the subject is thoroughly covered in other texts if nurses feel they are unsure of their own interviewing skills (Dickson *et al.*, 1997; Newell, 1994). Although they are considered to be beyond the specific remit of this book they are acknowledged as vital components in the overall teaching process.

Defining patients' needs or nursing diagnosis

Following patient assessment the next step is to identify each person's individual problems or needs. According to Castledine (1985), deciding the nature and priority of patients' problems is the most crucial stage of the teaching process. It is at this stage that nurses can demonstrate their clinical decision-making skills.

Kemp and Richardson (1994) suggest that where possible nurses should identify problems based on the assessment data and then consult the client to establish whether the nurse's interpretation of the data coincides with that of the patient. This reinforces to the patient that their views are important and it also helps ensure information has been interpreted correctly. For example, patients may prioritise information differently to nurses and it is important to gain their perception of their most important problems. The patient may identify something the nurse did not consider important or, indeed, the patient may say they are not troubled by an issue which a health professional may consider a problem. There is no need to identify problems which do not worry the patient if they do not affect the person's overall health.

Kemp and Richardson distinguish between a need and a problem as follows:

> Needs can be defined as something of necessity without necessarily being a problem. A patient's problem may be defined as something the patient cannot cope with which requires a solution.
>
> (1994: 31)

After identifying and verifying patients' problems the convention was to decide upon a goal which would contribute to resolution of the problem. As nursing diagnosis is a fashionable term these days it will be briefly discussed. A nursing diagnosis differs from a medical diagnosis in the following way:

> Areas of nursing diagnosis are related to, but distinct from medicine. Where medicine labels symptoms and pathology, nursing describes the effects of these symptoms and pathology on the activities and style of living now and in the future.
>
> (Little and Carnevali, 1976: 6)

According to Weber (1991) a nursing diagnosis is:

> A statement that describes the actual or potential health problems of a client based on a complete holistic assessment. The problem/s must be at least partially resolved through nursing interventions.
>
> (22)

A statement of a client problem

Refers to a health problem

Is based on objective and subjective assessment data

Is a statement of a nursing judgement

Is a short concise statement

Consists of a two-part statement (except that the 'related to' used within the NANDA* Taxonomy in Britain is commonly referred to as 'due to')

Is a condition that a nurse can prescribe care independently

Can be validated with the client.

Figure 4.4 Key components of a nursing diagnosis
Note: * North American Nursing Diagnosis Association

The key components of a nursing diagnosis, as suggested by Hogston (1997: 497) are illustrated in Figure 4.4.

There is considerable debate about whether diagnosis is a helpful move in nursing (Lutzen and Tishelman, 1996; Gordon, 1994; Booth, 1992; Webb, 1992). However, if the list in Figure 4.4 is carefully considered in relation to patient education it can be seen that there could be distinct practical advantages from aiming to be so specific. The use of a diagnosis is not to make nurses elitist or into mini-doctors, but it may help nurses to make a 'definitive statement from which the nurse determines a package of care for which she is accountable' (Hogston, 1997: 498).

If the science of patient education is to develop we must move away from broad, vague statements, the achievement of which cannot be evaluated. Therefore nursing diagnosis may facilitate educational development by using standardised, widely accepted diagnoses. This may enable studies to be more readily compared, which can then help increase the body of scientific knowledge on this subject. As was discussed in Chapter 2, in the past research studies have tended to be so disparate that they are difficult to compare. However, this assumption has yet to be tested. The potential advantage to be gained by using nursing diagnosis as outlined by Hogston (1997) is that it could help nurses to identify what they are doing for patients to give them greater delineation of their domain of practice.

The North American Nursing Diagnosis Association (NANDA) aims to define nursing problems and use a specified terminology to describe them and is a movement which has gathered weight over the past twenty years. This work is to promote a consensus of opinion in nursing and should facilitate standardisation of terms and understanding about nursing work. Imagine the chaos there would be in medicine if there was not a standard way of naming a problem such as an inflamed appendix. Unfortunately, with regard to patient teaching the only approved NANDA diagnosis relating directly to patient education in 1990 was that of *knowledge deficit*. So there are still large parts of patient education for which there is no NANDA approved terminology.

Nursing diagnosis can be used without using a NANDA approved diagnosis. The important point is that patients' unique needs are identified in a clear and comprehensive way in order that steps may be taken to solve the problem or alleviate the need. Whichever system is used the next step should be defining goals or, in educational terms, objectives should be set.

Goals

In patient education it is important that both the nurse and the patient/client are aware of what the goal of the teaching intervention will be. Only by knowing what both parties are aiming for is there any chance of success. In addition, only through objectively phrased goals can learning be evaluated. Goals setting will be influenced by the circumstances of each particular patient; if someone has physical disabilities such as poor vision or hearing difficulties it may influence interpretation of assessment data and the drafting of goals. Furthermore, if patients are involved in setting goals they may also serve as a form of motivation in the learning process. Negotiation with patients will offer best chances of success; patients will not do something just because they have been told to. Negotiation may be a brief discussion or more formally involving a contract, depending upon the patient teaching situation.

Goals must be realistic in terms of patients' situations and expectations, their likely length of contact with health professionals, the available resources and the abilities of the educators. When setting goals health professionals must strive to be realistic rather than to achieve the ideal (Fahrenfort, 1987). If diagnosis and setting of goals is incorrect all the remaining care will also be inappropriate. Thus, these steps are vital.

When setting goals and determining priorities for care it is also important to be practical and realistic regarding what nurses can reasonably be expected to deliver. It would be a waste of time to set goals which are beyond the nurses' capabilities. Similarly, in organisational managerial terms there must be provision made for nurses to be effective patient educators. As Luker and Caress (1989: 713) have quite rightly pointed out:

> it is unrealistic to exhort nurses to undertake assessments in order to formulate teaching strategies if one does not provide them with clear guidelines and the time and materials to act out the plan.

This is an important point and is a cautionary warning as there is little point in investing time setting goals which, due to constraints in the health care organisation, are unattainable.

According to the definition of patient education used in this book, in which the outcome of education is measured in behavioural change, many of the objectives of learning are couched in behavioural terms. However, as noted earlier, there are three types of learning, cognitive, affective and psychomotor, and learning goals could be phrased to reflect any of these types of learning. Examples of taxonomies of objectives for each domain of learning can be seen in Redman (1988) and may be helpful when deciding goals. However, in acute learning situations such a degree of precision may be over-ambitious. For nurses who have a specialist role in patient education the taxonomies may be helpful, but for most nurses in acute settings it is unlikely that these taxonomies would be used. Clearly, the nature of the objective should reflect the nature of the learning need or problem identified.

More pragmatically, consideration of the work of Maslow (1970) when setting learning objectives should help patients' needs be met in an appropriate hierarchical order. Goals relating to survival and safety needs must be met first. In acute care, learning objectives need to be restricted to what the patient can tolerate at the time. Some situations may preclude any teaching at all in the short term, but learning needs could be introduced to the care plan according to the patient's recovery. Some patients may be too ill to learn enough about their condition to be able to give informed consent

---

1   be patient focused: what the patient will achieve, do, learn, rather than what the nurse will do, demonstrate or teach.

2   reflect theoretical underpinnings which the nurse considers appropriate to the patient's needs.

3   be specific so that all involved parties know what is required. Vague goals will lead to vague teaching and may be impossible to evaluate.

4   they should have an identified time span.

5   the patient and the teacher and the family if relevant should have an unambiguous understanding of what is to be achieved.

6   the patient should have a say in determining objectives because health professionals and clients may have different priorities. If nurses aim to help patients achieve their goals they are more likely to succeed.

Figure 4.5 Key points when setting goals for patient education

for their treatment. In this case it may be appropriate to consider the learning needs of the patients' next of kin.

When setting goals or objectives the principles illustrated in Figure 4.5 should be borne in mind.

Conclusion

This chapter has explored issues surrounding the two related activities of assessment and planning prior to teaching in clinical settings with patients and clients. These two activities are prerequisites of any teaching intervention, however brief. In Chapter 5, we shall examine ways in which teaching can be put into practice. Finally, some suggestions for the evaluation of educational interventions will be outlined.

KEY POINTS FROM CHAPTER 4

1   *Patient education must be planned to suit the current health care climate* in which patients are in hospital for as short a stay as is possible. There is only a very limited amount of time in which patient education can occur. It must also be remembered

that while in hospital individuals may be so ill that education is not a priority. Shorter lengths of time in hospital plus acutely ill patients presents many challenges for those attempting to meet patients' educational needs.

2 *In order to make best use of any time* which is available it is advocated that patients' educational needs are assessed to help prevent time being wasted through inappropriate attempts at education and also to enable needs to be prioritised.

3 *It is important that nurses assess what each patient wants to know* because patients' and nurses' views and priorities have been found to differ.

4 *As patients' needs change* in response to changing health status, assessment must be ongoing.

5 *Assessment needs to take into account* the topics which patients wish to learn about, whether they are able to learn and the extent to which they wish to be involved and active in their care.

6 *The two main ways we can assess needs for education are through interview and observation.* The factors which may influence an assessment include age of patient, literacy, health status, and mental state.

7 *Once assessment data is available individuals' problems or needs must be identified.* Ideally these problems/needs should be verified with patients to ensure that the assessment data has been interpreted correctly. Recently, it has been fashionable to consider making a nursing diagnosis but this is still an area of great controversy in UK nursing circles.

8 *For each identified problem a goal must be set* which will facilitate its alleviation or resolution. Setting appropriate, precise goals will help to clarify the type of educational activity which is required. Goals must be realistic in relation to both the patients' and the nurses' abilities and resources.

9 *If attention is not paid to the above points patient education becomes a matter of pure chance.* Without clear and appropriate goals all subsequent care may be inappropriate, leading to wastage of nurses' and patients' time and resources. Successful, planned intervention depends to a large extent on the initial preparatory work mentioned in this chapter.

Chapter 5

Teaching strategies II: intervention and evaluation

Introduction

As we have seen in Chapter 4, assessment and planning are linked activities which prepare both nurse and patient for teaching and learning. The bulk of this chapter is concerned with strategies for *actual teaching* – in other words, the intervention phase, during which the nurse attempts, in collaboration with the patient, to put into practice the educational objectives she has defined and negotiated with the patient as a result of assessment and through the process of planning the educational experience. In a well-designed educational intervention, the patient is already enlisted as an active learner through these earlier processes, which 'set the scene' for what is to be taught. Similarly, planning is itself linked to the eventual evaluation of the extent of the success of the intervention, usually in terms of the patient's learning, and often is measured in terms of behaviour change. Like Chapter 4, this chapter attempts to offer guidance for the successful practice of educational interventions through reference to published research. The chapter also describes some barriers to effective patient education. Once again, it will be useful to consider the chapter in conjunction with the discussion of learning theories presented in Chapter 3.

Intervention

The form that the teaching and learning experience will take will vary according to each patient's situation and the approach adopted by health professionals. Skelton (1997) draws attention to the fact that whilst great store is set by patient-centred approaches, the practice of patient education often lags behind such ideals and is still dominated by a medical model approach. However, Skelton, as a result of her research regarding patients with lower back pain, suggests that the debate should not become polarised. Rather, patients and health professionals should negotiate their aims and this in turn will influence the teaching strategies used.

In addition teaching strategies will be affected by factors relating to nurses' place of work, which may be referred to as institutional factors. These will include time, resources (financial and personnel) and environmental factors (De Muth, 1989). Each of these will influence selection of teaching intervention. For example, what money is available to buy teaching aids such as videos and tapes, or to prepare and print information leaflets? What time have patients got to spend being taught, and where, in a clinical setting, is there a suitable place to teach patients and their families? Although many advocate a suitable place for patient teaching, how many wards or even hospitals and clinics can afford to have a dedicated teaching room?

Despite a body of research-based information which has been accumulating since the 1960s the effect of various teaching strategies is still unclear. The conclusion drawn by Theis and Johnson (1995) after conducting a substantial and thorough piece of research indicates that patient teaching tends to be on an *ad hoc* basis, using interventions of unknown effect and often with no positive, tangible outcomes: 'Although patient teaching has been an important role of the nurse for many years, it is still done in a random, often unstructured, manner' (Theis and Johnson, 1995: 100).

The intervention section of this chapter will comprise a résumé of verbal, written, audio-visual and computer-based teaching interventions; their associated strengths and weaknesses and points for good practice will be identified. According to a wide range of research presented in this chapter, it can be seen that a careful, planned approach is likely to yield greater success than an unplanned or random approach to education.

Acute situations

In acute hospital situations, because of a combination of institutional constraints, the physical and mental state of the patient and the need to attend to immediate physical safety needs, it may only be appropriate to supply information on a 'need to know' basis in order to promote basic survival and to enable informed consent to be given. However, there is research to suggest that even this may not always be achieved (Byrne *et al.*, 1988). In acute situations it will be important to keep instructions simple and to the point and be able to refer patients on for further information as required and when they are in a situation in which they are able to absorb further information (Ruzicki, 1989).

In an acute situation a verbal, one-to-one teaching session is likely to be the only feasible strategy, because patients may need to take a completely passive role. Leaving them to read leaflets, listen to tapes or watch videos will probably be too demanding for them.

Teaching interventions: verbal

Giving verbal information is one of the most widely used methods of patient education and this form of teaching intervention will be considered first. Ley (1982) examined the body of research-based literature concerning face-to-face interaction between hospital in-patients and health professionals for provision of information. Drawing from previous research on patients in medical, surgical and maternity units he reported that:

> The problem of patient dissatisfaction with communications is not limited to a given type of patient, nor is it limited to only one country. Nor is there any evidence in these survey results to suggest that the problem is decreasing as time passes.
>
> (340)

Looking at the problem from the professionals' expectations of the amount of information they wanted patients to possess, Ley reports (drawing primarily from the work of Hulka *et al.*, 1975a and 1975b) that the patients studied 'lacked about a third of the knowledge that their doctor wished them to have' (341).

One of the problems according to Ley is that patients are never given the information. Patients' perceptions about their lack of information and observational studies of what patients are told appear to confirm findings. The situation is further compounded by studies that illustrate that patients claim not to have understood what they are told.

Ley (1982: 348) reports that 'the majority of patients wish to know as much as possible about their illness, its causes, its treatment and its outcome'. More recently the Patient's Charter (D.o.H.,

1992) stated that patients have a right to full information about their treatment and their views should be taken into account before deciding about care. These goals can only be achieved through patient education.

To help clarify what information to offer patients he suggests the criteria listed in Figure 5.1 should be taken into account.

While it would be comforting to suggest that Ley's research is now rather outdated and that the situation has improved, more recent research illustrates that the problem is still evident. According to the Audit Commission (1993), which reports on an investigation into communication between patients and hospital staff, levels of communicated information were found to be inadequate. The report cites Whitehead (1993), who investigated the discharge procedures of 1000 patients. Just over 50 per cent replied and of these 35 per cent had not received any verbal advice or information when discharged. Such a low response rate is unfortunate as we are left

---

legal requirement: for example, Patient's Charter; informing patients, when prescribing medication, of the main risks of taking it, contra-indications and warning signs of problems arising.

patient's desires: as mentioned already and probably the most important criterion.

professional views: in some situations it may be decided that it is in the patient's best interests if information is withheld. This may cause a problem if the patient wishes to be informed.

behavioural objectives: in order for patients to undertake some activities, for example, regarding taking medication or modifying their diet, they must first know what to do.

rationality: patients must have enough information to make rational decisions about treatment.

empirical criteria: this concerns evidence to support the giving of information in terms of achieving a desired outcome or conversely the possibility that giving information will have a harmful effect.

Figure 5.1   Key points to help clarify the information to be offered to a patient

wondering about the views of the large number of people who did not respond.

With regard to clinical information, the Audit Commission draws attention to the importance of health professionals having good communication skills as one of the most crucial factors in the process. Patients reported that they experienced problems with the amount and content of the information received about their clinical care. Seven factors are given in the 1993 report as contributing to the quality of clinical communication:

1 *The amount of time for discussion*
This issue can be clearly illustrated by the following quotation:

> In the majority of urology clinics, men with a prostate problem are put on to the surgical waiting list after a consultation that on average lasts for seven minutes. In that time the patient is examined and he hears everything he is going to hear about his condition, treatment, the surgical procedure risks, and outcomes before he is admitted as an in-patient.
>
> (Audit Commission, 1993: 24–25)

Clearly, a seven-minute consultation would allow little, if any, time, for meaningful discussion. Yet it is on the basis of the interaction that the patient will agree (or not) to having a prostatectomy.

2 *Timing*
This refers to patients receiving information at the right time, rather than too late, at an inappropriate time or when too shocked to absorb it. They draw attention to the frequent occurrence of patients learning of the risks and complications of an operation, after the decision to operate has been taken, often just prior to signing the consent form. In the report it is suggested that this information should be given before the decision to operate is made.

3 *Conduct of consultations*
In the report the common practice of delivering information to people in vulnerable and probably pre-occupied circumstances was noted. For example, it was found that women referred to a surgical clinic with a breast lump were examined and had their entire consultation without being introduced to the doctor

conducting the examination. The woman was usually undressed, on the examination couch and covered only by a sheet. As the authors of the report suggest, this denies women their dignity and increases their vulnerability, which presumably reduces their ability to learn or retain the information given to them. Thus this trend is probably inefficient as well as improper.

4   *Support*
The unfortunate situation of people receiving bad news without a friend or relative with them to support them was found to be a common occurrence. However, the commissioners did report that in situations where a specialist nurse was present the degree of support available to patients was considerably greater.

5   *Contradictory messages*
Examples were given where conflicting information was given to patients. In the context of multi-professional team work the risks of this occurring increase. They cite the example of a woman being told a breast lump was 'nothing to worry about' by the surgeon, but that the radiotherapist mentioned the 'risk of recurrence'. Clearly, time needs to be spent to ensure that people have the opportunity of assimilating and checking all the information they are given.

6   *Uncertainty about who to ask for ongoing information*
Patients and relatives who need advice between scheduled hospital appointments reported that they did not know who to contact. The Commissioners found that often there was a process for gaining this information and advice but that the consumers were not aware of how to avail themselves of it.

7   *Confidentiality and the use of relatives to interpret*
This problem arose when patients did not speak English, but used relatives as interpreters. This raised an issue of confidentiality of patients' details and also that in some cases the 'interpreter' was a child and was an inappropriate representative.

Although the report did not focus upon the work of nurses in the communication process, indeed, surprisingly, nursing was hardly mentioned in the report at all, there are lessons to be learnt by all health professionals from the main findings presented above. In addition to which there is plenty of scope for nurses to help improve many of the aspects of communication difficulties mentioned.

As a result of the research presented above key points which need to be addressed when providing verbal information are included in Figure 5.2.

1   Introductions are important; if the patient does not already know the nurse, introductions should precede any teaching. Apart from knowing the nurse's name it is helpful if the patient understands his/her position and role and the remit of the teaching to be offered.

2   Some scheduled time should be allowed for the teaching.

3   The time when teaching is conducted is important and needs to be taken into account if the time allowed is to be used well.

4   The patient should not be in a vulnerable or powerless position when the teaching is conducted, for example, if the person is undressed or lying down they are at a psychological disadvantage during the interaction.

5   Include relatives in the teaching if appropriate because the patient can then 'go over' what they have been told with someone else who has heard exactly the same information. This can help clarify the information in addition to being a means of providing support.

6   The content of the information must be accurate and it is important that the messages are consistent between health professionals. Use of clinical guidelines and protocols are examples of how this may be achieved and will be discussed later.

7   Organise the process of giving information and ensure the patient and relatives are aware of the means by which they can get further information.

8   When a person does not speak English as a first language the use of an interpreter must be considered, although, of all the points listed above, this may be the most difficult to achieve as it is unlikely that a wide range of ethnic minority languages can be represented in each locality. However, it would seem reasonable for all ethnic groups which have a substantial representation in the local population to have on call, round-the-clock access to an interpreter.

Figure 5.2   Key points relating to the provision of verbal information arising from the Audit Commission (1993) report

While giving verbal information may be considered the simplest and easiest form of patient education it can be seen that it is a deceptively complex business. If patient education based on verbal instruction is to be successful it must be planned and structured.

Glimelius *et al.* (1995) investigated the importance that communication skills would have on patient education, especially the imparting of information. As a result of their work they recommend some practical tips to promote patient understanding of the information given to them (Figure 5.3). Although the research study concerned the needs of people with cancer, the information presented in Figure 5.3 would appear to be generally applicable. Many of the points made above would seem to be common sense but, as the research cited earlier indicates, many of these points are not regularly put into practice.

The message which emerges is that if part of the teaching intervention involves verbal communication it is important that nurses have appropriate communication skills to undertake this activity (Ley, 1982; Anderson and Sharpe, 1991; Faulkner *et al.*, 1991).

Teaching interventions: written

After verbal instruction great reliance is placed on the use of patient information sheets and leaflets by many health care professionals as a means of enhancing patient education. The rationale includes that patients do not remember all that they have been told, therefore written copy can endorse the verbal information (Beaver and Luker, 1997). Written material may be used to save time because patients can be left to read the information rather than a professional taking time to deliver it (a controversial point, as will be discussed later). Patient convenience may be enhanced as the information can be read when they want to rather than having to listen when a nurse has the time to talk. According to Coey (1996: 360) drawing from the work of Redman (1988) and Bernier (1993) the advantages of written material include that it is:

- reusable
- permanent
- readable at the reader's pace
- easy to reproduce
- easy to distribute

A. Communication
Prepare yourself physically and mentally
Create seclusion
Have an open attitude, pose open questions
Give emotional responses to emotional signals
Listen from the start of the talk
Respect silence
Use simple language
Encourage questions
Be honest

B. First information about serious disease

Before
Map the prerequisites
Create a relationship with the patient first
Plan the information
Invite a significant other to participate

During
Let the patient decide the speed
Be sincere
Give time for emotional reactions
Emphasise patient's own participation
Describe what will happen
Write down the most important information

Follow-up
Repeat the information
Ask the patient what he/she has comprehended
Teach the patient to ask questions
Be sensitive to emotional signals

C. General strategies for information
Give the most important information first
Give specific information, not just general
Use simple language with simple explanations
Try to structure the information, and tell the patient the structure
Remember that the patient can manage only a limited amount of information on the same occasion
Supplement verbal information with information written down during the talk
Ask the patient what he/she has understood

Figure 5.3   Key points to improve communication of information to patients
Source: Glimelius *et al.*, 1995: 173

- consistent in message conveyed
- portable

However, it is worth considering what makes a good information leaflet as the provision of written information alone will not enhance learning (Ley, 1982).

Many researchers have reported that written educational material is seriously flawed, often because the language is not suited to the reading ability of the consumer. Beaver and Luker (1997) report a survey in which the readability of 50 information booklets available to women with breast cancer in Britain was evaluated. They reveal that most booklets required a higher reading age than would be held by many such patients. Similarly Scriven and Tucker (1997) report the findings of a random sample of 27 hospitals in England regarding the quality and management of written information offered to women requiring hysterectomy. Not only do they report that for many women the information would be illegible, they also found that the timing of distributing the leaflets was on an *ad hoc* basis.

The work of Sarna and Ganley (1995) relating to patient education materials for people with lung cancer also led them to conclude that existing materials are inadequate and require advanced reading skills. Albert and Chadwick (1992) report inadequacies in patient information leaflets offered in general practice. They note that general practices have to follow guidelines specified by the government (D.o.H., 1989) when producing leaflets. They surveyed 85 practice leaflets and found that although the leaflets tended to be of good quality in terms of printing, in terms of simple, clear, communication there was room for improvement. They recommend using short sentences and short words, for example 'need' rather than 'require' or 'told' rather than 'notified'. They uphold the use of terms with which patients will be familiar, so terms such as 'acutely ill', 'continuity of care' or 'open access' are not recommended. Unnecessary words should be omitted. They advocate simple active sentences, for example 'A sees B' rather than 'B was seen by A'. They suggest using a personal writing style such as 'We (the doctors) believe' rather than 'The philosophy of this practice is ...'. Such advice appears to be applicable to other health care settings and should improve the quality of the literature from the reader's point of view.

The need for careful preparation of written material has been stressed by many others. The readability of written material has been widely investigated and the trend identified by research studies is that most educational material requires a reading level greater than the majority of patients possess (Hearth-Holmes *et al.*, 1997; Reed-Pierce and Cardinal, 1996; Davis *et al.*, 1994; Wells *et al.*, 1994; Davis *et al.*, 1993). In particular, meeting the needs of elderly people through written educational material needs careful consideration (Weiss *et al.*, 1995; Jackson *et al.*, 1994; Murphy *et al.*, 1993).

Reading ability can be measured using readability formulas such as the Gunning Frequency of Gobbledygook (FOG) Index (Gunning, 1968), the Simple Measure of Gobbledygook (SMOG) (McLaughlin, 1969) or the Flesch Formula (Flesch, 1974), two of which are illustrated in Figures 5.4 and 5.5.

Instruments such as those presented in Figures 5.4 and 5.5 can be useful when developing new educational leaflets. For example, Coey (1996) calculated the reading scores of three patient educational

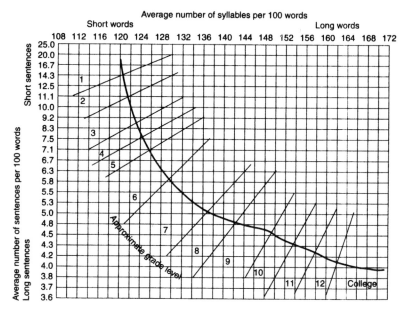

Figure 5.4   Gunning FOG Formula

Source: Adapted from Robert Gunning and Richard A. Kallan, *How to Take the Fog Out of Business Writing*, published by Dartnell, 1994. The FOG Index$_{SM}$ scale is a service mark licensed exclusively to RK Communications Consultants by D. and M. Mueller.

1. For short pieces, test the entire selection. For longer pieces, test at least three randomly selected samples of 100 words each. Do not use introductory paragraphs as part of the sample. Start each sample at the beginning of a paragraph.

2. Determine the average sentence length (*SL*) by counting the number of words in the sample and dividing by the number of sentences. Count as a sentence each independent unit of thought that is grammatically independent, that is, if its end is punctuated by a period, question mark, exclamation point, semicolon, or colon. In dialogue, count speech tags (e.g., 'he said') as part of the quoted sentence.

3. Determine the word length (*WL*) by counting all the syllables in the sample as if reading the words aloud. Divide the syllables by the number of words in the sample and multiply by 100.

4. These indices are then applied to the formula to compute the reading ease,

$$RE = 206.835 - 1.015\ SL - 0.846\ WL$$

where *RE* is the reading ease score, *SL* is the average sentence length in words, and *WL* is the average word length measured as syllables per 100 words.

Interpretation of the Flesch reading ease score

Reading ease	Grade	Description of style	No. syllables 100 words	Average sentence length
90–100	5	Very easy	123	8
80–90	6	Easy	131	11
70–80	7	Fairly easy	139	14
60–70	8–9	Standard	147	17
50–60	10–12	Fairly difficult	155	21
30–50	College	Difficult	167	25
0–30	College graduate	Very difficult	192	29

Source: Flesch, 1974: 184–186, 247–251

Figure 5.5 Flesch Formula

leaflets on stoma care using the FOG index and found that only about 40 per cent of the UK population were likely to understand them. Mumford (1997) presents a very useful analysis of the application of readability formulae to written materials designed by nurses. She identifies associated strengths and weaknesses and makes seven very pertinent recommendations including exploring why nurses produce leaflets, and studying variables in health settings that affect leaflet comprehension.

Readability is also not the only point to take into account. Several reports have acknowledged that a substantial portion of the population have low literacy skills or may be illiterate (Mayeaux *et al.*, 1996). When providing patient education there is also, then, the need to check whether patients can read. As Dollahite *et al.* (1996: 123) rather succinctly put it:

> Many of the publications reviewed can be read and understood by many Americans but there were few for the millions that have limited literacy skills.

Another factor to bear in mind is that patients' cultural background may be different from that of the people who prepared the information and it is important that this does not impede its use (Wilson, 1996). English may not be the patient's first language, in which case translated versions will be needed.

Furthermore, whilst it is important that reading ability is taken into account there are also other factors which help to make written educational material effective, such as size of font, use of white space, colour and cartoons. Coey (1996) recommends that a font size of 12 is preferable to that of 10; illustrations should be near to relevant text; white space between text makes reading easier as does matt paper and black print on white paper. Overall, she recommends that the information should be as short as possible without losing the sense and meaning it is designed to convey.

An interesting study was conducted by Reid *et al.* (1995: 32) to:

1   determine what and how much persons with diabetes could recall immediately after reading a pamphlet,
2   identify text and reader characteristics that may influence recall (and thus suggest guidelines for writing educational material),
3   determine whether what the reader wanted to know agreed with what a physician thought the reader should know.

Using a 1000-word extract from a widely used diabetes pamphlet and a sample of 28 adults with diabetes they investigated reader recall, text and reader characteristics. They found that recall was low despite it being tested straight after the pamphlet was read; an average of only 8 out of 108 items were recalled from the pamphlet. Of the 73 sentences in the pamphlet, 40 were deemed to be poorly constructed according to the criteria used. Number of years at school correlated with number of items recalled (less schooling relating to fewer items). People with higher vocabularies recalled more ideas. Prior knowledge had a positive correlation with number of items recalled. Less than a third of the sample identified the same items as the physicians as being most important, illustrating that it cannot be assumed that professionals and staff interpret the information in the same way.

As a result of this study the authors concluded that whilst readability of the pamphlet was an important point there are also other features of the text which educators should bear in mind when producing educational material:

> Some researchers suggest that educational material will be easier to understand if authors follow guidelines from readability formulas and use shorter words and sentences. This is not our position.
>
> (Reid *et al.*, 1995: 35)

They suggest that the points illustrated in Figure 5.6 should be taken into account (in addition to readability) when developing written educational materials in order to promote recall of the information. They also recommend the linking of old information to new, for example 'Your mother taught you to eat fruits and vegetables. She was right' (ibid., 36). This would be in keeping with cognitive learning theory in which it is suggested that new material should be presented in a way that builds on existing knowledge.

Higgins and Ambrose (1995) noted from the literature that written educational material had been found to have more effect when adjunct questions are included. Adjunct questions are those set within the written material, say at the beginning, middle and end and are designed to help focus thoughts and help people retain the material. Thus they investigated the effect of adding adjunct questions to written material on the learning of older people who needed cataract surgery.

Use familiar words:	jargon should not be included.
Use organisers:	list key points to be discussed; case studies, stories or examples can be used to introduce a point.
Use signallers:	tell the reader the structure of the information; include transition sentences from one point to another; write summary statements or paragraphs.
Insert questions into the information:	e.g. before the information to focus the reader's attention (referred to as adjunct questions by some); within the material to help the reader at the point of initial learning; at the end to help recall.

Repeat the main points to enhance recall.

Encourage the reader to develop his/her reading and self-monitoring skills.

Figure 5.6   Key points to enhance recall of written information
Source: Reid *et al.*, 1995

An experimental treatment group, a control treatment group and a control group were set up. The experimental group received a booklet with additional questions, such as, 'Think about the forthcoming surgery: why is it a risk? What is the greatest risk? How long does it take to heal completely?'

The treatment control group received the same material in similar booklet form but did not have adjunct questions included. The control group did not receive any booklet. A sample of 90 participants with a mean age of 77 years was involved. Although both groups receiving the booklet scored significantly higher than those who did not, the people in the experimental group did not do any better than those in the treatment control group, but the patients did report that the questions were useful and helped them.

The authors therefore concluded that the use of adjunct questions did not improve cognitive recall of the information, which they found puzzling in view of the strong support expressed for the questions by the group members. Rather surprisingly, they did not question the wisdom of using a written medium for people requiring eye surgery. However, of importance is the fact that the authors did not just presume that the addition of adjunct questions would be useful. They set up a rigorously controlled experiment to enable them to evaluate the impact of the intervention. More of this type of work should be conducted.

As a result of their research Scriven and Tucker (1997) make the recommendations listed in Figure 5.7, which build upon those of Reid *et al.* (1995) to improve existing practice regarding written information.

Although there is a large volume of research berating the shortcomings of written educational material there is research to illustrate that it can be effective (Butow *et al.*, 1998; Fitzgerald and Glotzer,

---

1   Authors of leaflets should obtain professional advice on layout and design of leaflets.

2   Authors of leaflets should refer to past patients to ensure that the information is relevant to the intended target group.

3   The advice should be realistic in its assessment of the likelihood of potential problems/side effects.

4   Evaluation of leaflets should be undertaken, rather than assumptions made about their usefulness.

5   The dissemination of written information should be undertaken in a co-ordinated manner, such that patients receive literature at the appropriate time and staff know who is responsible for its dissemination.

6   Authors should critically assess their work to ensure it does not implicitly support gender stereotypical behaviour which may alienate a section of the readers.

7   Advice should be framed in such a way that the reader feels empowered rather than undermined.

8   Information should be given about why particular advice (e.g. about lifting) is considered important.

Figure 5.7   Key points to enhance the presentation of written information
Source: Scriven and Tucker, 1997: 113

1995; Bernier, 1993; Weinman, 1990; Edwards, 1990; Gibbs *et al.*, 1989; Ley, 1982).

For example, Frederikson and Bull (1995) used a patient education leaflet to help patients have a more active role in their care. Eighty patients who were consulting their doctor during normal surgery hours were involved. A single sheet leaflet was used to explain to patients what constituted a 'good consultation' to make communication between doctor and patient clearer and the interaction more effective. The leaflet explained how patients could be more involved, how to organise what they wanted to say, and encouraged them to ask questions rather than just recite symptoms. A quasi-experimental approach was used in which experimental patients were given the leaflet and the controls were not. The doctor was 'blind' to the membership of the groups and subjectively rated all patients on the extent to which he considered the consultation to be 'good', 'average' or 'poor'. There were 'clear differences between the control and experimental groups in terms of the proportion of consultations being perceived as good, average or poor' (54). The authors state that the sample was relatively small and that greater experimental work is required, but as an initial exploratory study the results were very encouraging. The leaflet used is illustrated in Figure 5.8 because its simplicity is a good example of the positive effect that can be gained from well produced material.

From the research presented in Figure 5.8 it can be deduced that the production of an effective information leaflet is not necessarily a simple, cheap alternative to personal one-to-one teaching, to be used to save nurses' time. Mumford (1997) concludes her article on the production of written information leaflets with a cautionary quotation from the Associate Editor of the British Medical Journal, who, after discussing the poor quality of patient information leaflets, warns:

> Does all that sound difficult? Time consuming? Expensive? It is, and that's why so much that is given to patients is so awful.
> (Smith, 1992: 1242; cited by Mumford, 1997)

Teaching interventions: audio and audio-visual

A third method of teaching intervention is that based on the use of audio-visual material (Barber *et al.*, 1995). Many people now have equipment that would enable them to listen to tapes or watch videos at home, and hospital and health care settings also have such

STOP	before you go in to see the doctor we would like you to take time to go through the following points.
THINK	about why you have come to see the doctor today. — what is wrong — what is troubling you — what you think the problem is — what is worrying you about your health — and what you hope the doctor can do for you.
TELL	the doctor all of these things as clearly and concisely as possible right at the beginning of the consultation. DON'T leave important points till you are about to leave.
LISTEN	to what the doctor has to say as well. If you need more information – ask. The doctor is happy to explain things but you need to indicate what it is that you want to know.
REMEMBER	the doctor is not a mind reader and relies on you to: STOP THINK & TELL

Figure 5.8   An example of an information leaflet which was found to be effective
Source: Frederikson and Bull, 1995: 56

resources; therefore widespread use of tapes and videos has become a widely exploited teaching medium.

The advantages include that they can be prepared or acquired in advance and the patient and nurse can decide the most appropriate time to use them. The colour, sound and animation offer an opportunity for a stimulating and varied teaching medium. They can provide continuity of education which is started in hospital and then reinforced through use at home. Carers and families can also be educated using audio-visual aids. Dalayon (1994) reports that patients rated video presentation as the most useful teaching strategy, although it was found that the nurses preferred demonstrations.

The disadvantages include that they may be substituted for personal teaching delivered by a health professional. Thus the patient is asked, for example, to watch a video on pre-operative preparation rather than having a personal meeting and discussing the subject face to face. These aids may provide a rather general covering of the subject rather than an individualised approach. For example, the commentator's voice is often without any accent or perhaps a very cultured, well spoken accent to which many people from the provinces would not relate. Dietary advice may not reflect local foodstuffs and habits or the hospital and health care team may be unfamiliar to many patients. Thus the actual content may be accurate but the patient is less likely to relate it to their own experiences. Expense, resources and provision of a suitable environment to listen to or view the material may also be a problem for some. Both strengths and weaknesses identified above have been verified through research, as will be discussed below.

Nathan *et al.* (1994) investigated whether patients were interested in having their consultation with their doctor tape-recorded so that they could listen to it later or let their relatives hear exactly what they had been told. From a sample of 425 people, 257 participated in the survey and 54 per cent thought they would find a recording helpful; 60 per cent thought relatives would listen to it and 85 per cent said they were prepared to bring a blank tape with them. However, as the authors themselves state, the study did not extend to examine whether recorded consultations would lead to improved compliance with treatment. Thus the idea was well received but empirical work would be required to examine whether the initiative could lead to improved health outcomes.

Agre *et al.* (1994) conducted a randomised controlled trial using videotape to present information to patients about colonoscopy prior to them giving consent to the procedure. Informed consent is a vital step in patient care but the best way to inform patients and the amount of information required have not been widely studied. The objectives were to:

1   investigate whether presenting information on videotape could improve knowledge and if this could be improved through a discussion with their doctor, and
2   investigate whether increased knowledge led to increased anxiety about the procedure.

(272)

Of the 224 patients approached, 201 agreed to participate. Patients were randomised into three groups, those receiving video and discussion, those receiving video only and those receiving discussion. All were asked to complete the State Trait Anxiety Inventory to assess levels of anxiety and all completed a short multiple choice questionnaire to assess their knowledge and understanding of colonoscopy.

As a result of this work the authors recommend a two-part disclosure process. Using a videotape ensured that all patients received the same information, which helped provide consistency and clarity of information presented. The video could be played repeatedly and started and stopped at the patients' convenience. If this were done prior to the consultation it would give people time to think about issues and ask for further clarity or information, thus helping promote discussion.

The results of this study thus support the value of audio-visual material in patient education, as did the study by O'Donnell *et al.* (1995), who investigated the use of video-based sexually transmitted disease patient education for its impact on condom acquisition. They found that: 'condom acquisition almost doubled with the use of culturally appropriate, video-based intervention' (817).

Wicklin and Foster (1994) investigated whether, and in what way, a videotape could be used to help reduce pre-operative anxiety in patients who were to have same-day surgery. The authors used two different videos. In one a nurse described the scenario of procedures for same-day surgery patients. In the other, similar information was presented but from the patient's perspective, the situation as if seen through the eyes of a patient. Thus the information to be conveyed was the same but the educational approach was different. According to the results there was no difference in perceived anxiety between the groups, indicating that the personalised approach did not significantly decrease anxiety scores. However, the authors felt that this result should not be interpreted as the video having no value but that further work in this area of developing educational initiatives should be undertaken.

In a study by Powell and Edgren (1995), educational videotapes were mailed to a sample of patients to help improve compliance with medication in an experimental study involving 4246 people. The subjects were divided into an experimental and a control group. However, no difference in compliance with medications was detected as a result of the initiative. The results of this study suggest that videos must be used in addition to other educational interventions. A single intervention does not seem to change behaviour.

It is unlikely that simply giving a patient a video and leaving them to watch it will be an effective means of education on its own. However, appropriately selected videos may form a useful part of a planned broad teaching strategy.

Bartlett (1990) discusses the use of the telephone as an educational medium. On one hand the telephone presents numerous communication problems in that non-verbal communication (often a substantial part of our message) is lost, and it demands good listening skills. However, telephones can also be a valuable means of education (Radecki et al., 1989; Mahoney et al., 1983; Stirewalt et al., 1982; Meissner, 1990). From the literature reviewed Bartlett (1990: 216) suggests that the telephone could be used to improve teaching opportunities in the following ways:

- Patients discharged from hospital could be telephoned routinely to assess their progress.
- Persons with chronic illnesses such as diabetes, asthma or epilepsy should be able to call for advice at any time of the day, especially in acute situations.

As such there is scope for development of the telephone in patient education.

Teaching interventions: using computers

A fourth means of delivering educational material is via the use of information technology and this will be briefly discussed in this section. According to Kahn (1993) there are four main types of computer-based patient education, as illustrated in Figure 5.9.

When appraising the accomplishments of computer-based learning Kahn suggests:

> At virtually all levels of education the interactive computer is at least as effective as traditional teaching methods.
>
> (93)

He believes that computers may be more available than people who always have other responsibilities; they can be infinitely patient and consistent; they can facilitate individual learning as people can work at their own pace; they can be particularly useful for people who need to learn about a sensitive or embarrassing subject; and in

1   *Drill and practice*: to solve problems or answer multiple-choice type questions. Feedback can be offered until the user can demonstrate the correct knowledge.

2   *Tutorials*: in which textual information is presented to the patient who is then asked questions about it. Follow-up in terms of revisiting sections or getting greater detail about selected associated topics can be given.

3   *Simulations and games*: are a more sophisticated level of computer technology and can be used to encourage patient learning. Simulations enable the patient to make decisions in a safe environment. They can learn from their mistakes as the computer will be able to judge whether their response was correct or not. Games can involve fantasy and fun and may make learning a more enjoyable experience for some people.

4   *Artificial reality*: is similar to games and simulations but involves greater use of advanced computing technology involving three-dimensional graphics, sound, and using hoods, goggles or gloves to introduce tactile simulations.

Figure 5.9 The four main types of computer-based patient education
Source: Kahn, 1993

addition feedback can be given and the whole process documented. In principle these advantages are laudable. However, to achieve a programme of this sophistication requires considerable computing expertise. Kahn (1993) cites many examples of studies where computer-based learning has been a successful intervention (Wetstone *et al.*, 1985; Dearoff, 1986; Rippey *et al.*, 1987; Leirer *et al.*, 1988; Jimison *et al.*, 1992).

Other computing techniques which have great potential in terms of patient education include multi-media computing, in which computers are linked to videos or compact discs. Developments such as using touch-screens instead of a keyboard will help improve the acceptability of highly technical mediums to people who are not particularly computer literate (Glasgow *et al.*, 1997). Luker and Caress (1991), for example, report that a keyboard can be modified to help simplify its use.

Skinner *et al.* (1993) consider the evolution of computer-based education programmes from the early programmes which have been referred to as 'electronic page turners'. They were based on text which patients were asked to read and they were then given appropriate questions to answer. Thus they covered material that had previously been contained in written format. More recently more individualised patient education has been achieved to couple the advantages of a personalised approach with the efficiency of computerised material. Sophisticated computer-based packages can gather information from the patient, involve it in the educational material and thus adapt material as though a one-to-one encounter was taking place.

The value of personalised teaching material was tested by Osman *et al.* (1994), who conducted a randomised controlled trial involving 801 patients with asthma. The subjects were randomised into a control group receiving conventional outpatient education at the clinic or surgery. The experimental group received the conventional information plus four printed booklets on asthma management which were personalised to their medication and needs using an existing computerised database. The information focused on the management of asthma rather than clinical information about the condition. The authors report that after a year patients in the experimental group had greater understanding of their condition and how to control it and their hospital admission rates had been reduced by 51 per cent. The authors concluded that:

> The use of a computer to integrate education material with personal management plans was important to the success of this programme. This allowed a large and rather impersonal intervention to take on some of the features of a small group management programme in linking education to personal management.
>
> (Osman *et al.*, 1994: 571)

The potential benefits of computer-assisted learning (CAL) packages for patients needing continuous ambulatory peritoneal dialysis are discussed by Luker and Caress (1991). They suggest that CAL packages meet several important criteria when supplying additional teaching opportunities. For example, CAL packages can be used as an additional teaching intervention rather than as a substitute for any existing intervention, a point which was supported by the work of Krishna *et al.* (1997). Luker and Caress claim that CAL can be readily accessible to patients, irrespective of the presence of a nurse.

This of course is a debatable point depending upon the facilities of the health care environment and the degree of computer literacy possessed by the patients. The package should be self-directing to allow patients to work at their own pace. They suggest that there should be novelty and stimulation value over and above that of existing learning materials. Finally, they mention that feedback should be provided to the patient by the CAL package.

Luker and Caress (1989) report that computer-based learning was found to be acceptable to older people, who may often be assumed to be the people who may have most difficulty with this medium (Rippey *et al.*, 1987). Dearoff (1986) also reports that computer-based learning was well received, that patients can work at their own pace, they may have control of their learning, they can repeat sections without embarrassment and that computers can be adapted to allow for people with some disabilities. Computers can help people with literacy problems, and graphics and sound can be used to help convey information.

As information technology develops, more sophisticated educational packages become possible. For example, Buchanan *et al.* (1995) investigated the use of an intelligent interactive system to deliver individualised information to patients. The package was in two parts: first, an interactive history-taking section in which patients who had migraine were assessed; second, an interactive explanation tailored to individual needs was developed. The package was developed because doctors in the USA are not able, due to financial constraints on their time, to spend much time communicating with patients. If an effective artificial intelligence system could be developed then physician time could be saved. The system was still being developed when reported, using very small samples, of 3 and 16 people, and while the feedback about greater information about migraine headaches was largely positive, further work and testing was still to be conducted. Such work is still under development but gives us a glimpse of the potential that sophisticated computer-based teaching interventions could offer in the future.

The Internet is a further educational resource which is now opening up. Smith (1998) offers useful advice to health professionals when he suggests that patient education sites should be checked before they are recommended to patients in case they have been developed by organisations which introduce a bias into the material or have commercial interests in the topic. He also points out that we need to be aware that:

Many web sites contain copyrighted information (even though this may not be specifically stated) and as such the information cannot be downloaded, printed, or distributed without the owner's consent. On the other hand, direct viewing of free sites is legal, and can be a valuable means of keeping patients informed.

(12)

He concludes his article with a list of potentially valuable web sites which may be suitable for patient education. It can be anticipated that the Internet will become a powerful means of patient education in the next century. It is important that nurses start to become familiar with the quality and range of material on the web. Patients who are computer literate and who have access to 'on-line' facilities will be in a position to race ahead of nurses in terms of awareness of the resources available to them via the web. The Internet will open up vast sources of information, albeit for relatively small numbers of patients. For the first time patients are gaining access to state-of-the-art information in their own homes and health care professionals are not the gate-keepers to this resource, which will add a new and interesting dimension to patient education.

Telematics is a rapidly expanding area and refers to the use of providing information from a remote computer to patients who are able to access it locally via their television or computer using telecommunications links. This is an important area of development in patient education but its potential has yet to be tested in practice. At present the concept of telematics is still an intervention for the future, but in the next millennium it is expected that it will have a significant role to play in the education of patients and their relatives. Bearing in mind that it is anticipated that we will be doing our shopping via telematic links before too long it is reasonable to assume that patient education will be delivered via this medium some day. However, as the infrastructure is not yet in place it is not undertaken in anything other than an experimental capacity at present.

Even so, Lewis (1996) conducted an interesting study which also serves to keep the state of computer-based learning in perspective. She investigated what patient educators themselves felt about using computer-based patient education. Involving a sample of 300 certificated diabetes educators in America, she found that while the educators were interested in computer-based patient education as an educational tool, the majority were not currently using it. The main reasons for this were:

- lack of computer availability for patients
- limited financial resources
- lack of time for patients to learn computing skills
- limited availability of computers for educators
- limited computer training for educators
- limited availability of educational software.

As America is considered amongst the most computer literate nations in the world, these findings are probably even more applicable to many other countries. This study helps remind us that currently we are seeing only the potential of computers in patient education rather than the reality.

Psychomotor skills

When planning this book it was envisaged that there would be a substantial section on teaching patients psychomotor skills. Surprisingly, extensive computer-based searches of nursing, medical and psychology databases have failed to unearth research-based evidence on this topic. Whilst there is no shortage of material on relatively new teaching interventions involving computers, the more mundane, but fundamental topic of psychomotor skill development is under-resourced in the literature. Nurses spend considerable amounts of time teaching patients skills, but there is a dearth of material to illuminate good practice. For example, what is the best way to teach an individual how to change a stoma bag, to use an inhaler, to give an injection or to self-administer oxygen? Many of the key *general* educational skills are doubtless relevant to verbal and written skills development. However, the paucity of information is most acutely felt in relation to giving a demonstration, being a role model, the impact of learning styles upon the acquisition of psychomotor skills, how well a demonstration would work relative to showing the patient a video. To take a single instance, the use of modelling is a mainstay of some psychotherapeutic work (Bandura, 1977) and is of proven efficacy. Yet no studies which explicitly explore the role of modelling in patient education have been found in the literature.

Some information is available in relation to other professions, such as how to train a surgeon to perform micro-surgery, but not in relation to patient education. This would appear to be an area of nursing practice which is in urgent need of attention. Personal experience in patient teaching suggests that the points in Figure 5.10 are important.

Set aside enough, uninterrupted time in which to complete the demonstration.

Do the demonstration in a suitable environment.

Have all the necessary equipment close to hand.

Have spares of all equipment in case the demonstration does not work at first or it may need to be repeated.

Engage the patient's attention.

Explain verbally what you will do and why.

Do the demonstration.

Go over each stage of the demonstration either verbally or in actions as a recap.

Have the patient shadow (mime) each stage in the demonstration.

Ask the patient what they thought were the key points of the demonstration.

Arrange with the patient when they wish to have a repeat demonstration.

Negotiate when they will do the skill under supervision.

Ensure that this is as close to the time of the demonstration as possible.

Ensure that time is made available for repeated practice with feedback and reinforcement.

Check whether they wish a family member/friend to be taught the skill.

Use leaflets/videos or other available resources to augment the demonstration.

Figure 5.10 Suggestions for demonstrating a psychomotor skill

The points in Figure 5.10 may be of use but are basically anecdotal. What could a controlled research study add? Let us examine a couple of examples of possible gains from clear studies of the components of psychomotor teaching in patient education. Patient attention is not inexhaustible. As a result, it may be that repetition of a demonstration, contrary to our intuition, does not enhance learning, since inattention creeps in. Moreover, repetition takes time, which could be employed by both nurse and patient in some other pursuit. In the case of the nurse, this time also has a cost implication. Thus, a study comparing different numbers of repetitions of a demonstration would potentially be valuable. Similarly, we are told that 'practice makes perfect', yet it is well demonstrated in the psychology literature that some types of task performance improve more readily with massed practice, whilst others respond better to spaced practice. An examination of the different effects of massed and spaced practice in teaching psychomotor skills to patients would be welcome. Indeed, it might be that many such studies, each looking at a different category of task, would be useful.

Selection of teaching intervention

From the above discussion it can be seen that there are a variety of teaching modes which can be used to facilitate education. It is up to each nurse's judgement, guided where possible by empirical evidence, to decide which approach is most suited to her/his client group and working environment. This decision will clearly be influenced by issues such as time available for nurses to spend on teaching and amount of time patients have available for learning. Resources and facilities, patients' and nurses' abilities will also play a part. As a profession we still lack hard evidence about which are the most useful strategies to adopt in particular educational situations (Chapman *et al.*, 1995) although a growing body of research-based evidence is now available.

Another important factor is that the degree of control that nurses can exert over the patient environment is often rather limited. Luker and Caress (1989) mention that due to current health care constraints, in which nurses have little influence upon length of hospital stay or time of discharge, it can be difficult for nurses to deliver planned teaching. This is a point which will be returned to in Chapter 8.

Theis and Johnson (1995) conducted a meta-analysis of the results of studies which had evaluated the impact of strategies for teaching patients. They included 73 studies which met their inclusion criteria. Analysis is based on 'effect sizes' which are calculated for each study as follows:

$$\text{Effect size} = \frac{\text{treatment group mean} - \text{the control group mean}}{\text{within group standard deviation}}$$

In this way the results of studies which are comparable in terms of design are 'pooled' and the overall trends within the data are measured. This approach synthesises the results of many individual studies and thus can calculate the impact of a number of studies rather than considering a series of similar studies in isolation. However, the studies must have been investigating the same variables in order to compare 'like with like'. Going back to the points raised in Chapter 2, it is vital that variables and methods are clearly defined so that future consumers of research can grasp exactly what was done. Meta-analysis can only be conducted if the primary studies are unambiguously presented.

The following conclusions were drawn according to the best effect sizes in terms of being the most advantageous to learning outcomes.

1   Structured teaching (i.e., planned teaching is much more effective than a random question and answer session with the patient).
2   Reinforcement of teaching is crucial.
3   Independent study packages – these appeared to be beneficial but further work is required.
4   Use of multiple strategies is to be recommended.

A most important finding was that:

> 66% of the subjects who received planned patient teaching had better outcomes than did control group subjects who received routine care.
>
> (Theis and Johnson, 1995: 102)

Another very important result was that verbal teaching was found to be the *least* effective intervention of those examined, despite its being amongst the most common forms of teaching. It would appear that if a simple verbal teaching intervention is used it needs to be combined with other interventions if patient outcomes are to be enhanced. For example, they report that the use of alternative methods such as audio-visual aids or written material improved the learning outcomes of 65 per cent of the people in the experimental groups. Thus they would appear to be a useful strategy in addition to other methods, as once produced they can be used repeatedly with little extra work.

Theis and Johnson found that the use of independent study packages had a positive effect upon learning, but as only a small number of studies using this means of education were included in their analysis further research is needed.

They conclude their report by stating:

> Nurse clinicians owe it to their patients to provide them with teaching strategies that provide the best results, while being cost effective to produce and use.
>
> (104)

Their findings support the advice offered by Ruzicki (1989), who recommends whenever possible the use of a pre-developed structured programme with ready prepared audio-visual aids, and supporting literature. This, she argues, would save nurses the pressure of having to develop teaching objectives and prepare a programme for all patients. However, she also accepts that it will not be possible to have a structured teaching programme for every patient and for those with less commonly encountered educational needs. For such patients Ruzicki suggests nurses draw from their own pool of knowledge and use reference books as appropriate.

Mullen and Green (1990) reviewed literature on educational and behavioural interventions in clinical preventive medicine (and so their review is perhaps an analysis of health education rather than patient education) and came to two major general conclusions:

1   No single educational approach is better than any other.
2   The effectiveness of specific interventions depends on their appropriate selection and application.

(475)

As a result of a meta-analysis of 102 studies concerning education to enable patients to follow prescribed medication regimens, Mullen and Green confirmed that five well-known educational principles were found to influence the effectiveness of patient teaching. They were:

- *Reinforcement* – praise for achievement of a goal.
- *Feedback* – informing the patient on their progress towards achieving goals. They suggest that for long-term goals any way of showing patients their progress may be used as a means of communicating feedback.
- *Individualisation* – giving patients the chance to set the pace of their learning and to ask questions. They suggest that this requires more than saying 'Have you any questions?' at the end of an interaction. It may be the use of interview sessions or telephone help lines. Alternatively it may be combining a mix of strategies to suit an individual, for example, some verbal information, plus leaflets and a video to watch when at home. However, they warn that the use of a combination of approaches must be in addition to personal contact rather than a replacement for it.
- *Facilitation* – this involves helping patients to achieve their goals such as making a new action more memorable by pairing a new behaviour with a usual routine or altering a habit to enable a new action to be accommodated more readily, or conversely, helping a person to avoid barriers to taking action, thus helping them to put advice or information into action.
- *Relevance* – the learning process is more likely to be successful if the individual perceives it to be relevant to their own situation and interests. Thus a thorough assessment of the patient prior to undertaking patient education will enhance the chances of success because the educator will have a better understanding of what will be most relevant to the patient. Mullen and Green suggest that it is lack of this interaction that may undermine the possible success of leaflets or videos which do not relate to a patient specifically. In such circumstances it is important that the educator takes the time to illustrate how the information to be read or viewed is relevant to them personally.

A further meta-analysis was conducted by Mullen *et al.* (1992) on research relating to education of patients with cardiac problems. They found that the 'channels of communication used' such as media plus personal communication, or one-to-one communication alone did not influence the outcome, but that adherence to the educational principles (reinforcement, feedback etc.) did affect outcome. Whilst they report that there were no differences in outcome related to total hours of contact time or number of contacts, they conclude that it is not the amount of time spent with a patient *per se* which is important, rather it is the way in which the time is used.

When considering the efficacy of teaching interventions, Haynes *et al.* (1987) reviewed literature to help clarify which educational interventions were most likely to help patients continue to take their medications. Defining short-term as less than two weeks they identify the following factors as influential teaching strategies:

For all regimens
Information:
1   keep the prescription as simple as possible
2   give clear instructions on the exact treatment regimen, preferably written

For long-term regimens
Reminders:
3   call if appointment missed
4   prescribe medication in concert with patient's daily schedule
5   stress importance of compliance at each visit;
6   titrate frequency of visits to compliance need

Rewards:
7   recognise patient's efforts to comply at each visit; decrease visit frequency if compliance high

Social support:
8   involve patient's spouse or other partner

If the points made above are applicable to nurses' client groups, their adoption into teaching strategies will help nurses to incorporate research-based information into their own teaching standards.

Haynes *et al.* (1987) acknowledge that simply informing practitioners about good practice is not enough to ensure that it is adopted. They stress the need for applying proven techniques of continuing education such as audit of performance, and feedback from deviations from expected standards of care and appropriate training of future educators (165). These issues are known to be crucially important to the success of patient education and will be discussed in more detail in Chapter 8 of this book.

Structure of the educational intervention

Whatever teaching techniques are selected, the way they are used and the overall structure of the educational intervention is important. This does not mean that the intervention must be elaborate or time-consuming, but it does mean that the overall package of education should be thought out rather than offered in a random way. The protocol for many other forms of patient care is planned and known in advance, and education need be no different. For example, from the onset it is worth deciding if a patient will require any special learning materials such as pamphlets, videotapes or referral to a particular specialist, such as a pharmacist or clinical nurse specialist or peer support group. Such interventions can be planned in advance even if it is known that the patient will not use them immediately. In this way it may save a last-minute rush when the patient is on the point of discharge (Bubela *et al.*, 1990).

Continuity of patient education after discharge may be improved if referrals are made to community health care agencies or support groups. Community referrals must include an outline of what information was given and suggestions for future education.

Bostrom *et al.* (1994), whose research was outlined in Chapter 4, suggest the following practice implications arising from their research:

1   Discharge instructions for patients hospitalised on general medical and surgical units should focus on medications, treatments and complications and enhancing quality of life.
2   Nurses and other health care providers must take a proactive role in providing patient education because patients underestimate their post-discharge learning needs during hospitalisation.
3   One or more mechanisms are necessary as patients re-evaluate learning needs after they return home from the hospital.

(88)

As hospitals endeavour to provide the highest quality of patient care at the lowest possible cost, understanding the continuum of patient care that exists between the hospital and community is critical. Ideally, nurses should strive for an 'unbroken' or seamless continuum of patient care that would address patient learning needs both during and after hospitalisation.

(89)

No-one would dispute the importance of continuity of education as patient situations change, but to provide a 'seamless' education service a great deal of preparation is required in terms of liaison, communication and documenting of information.

Evaluation

The final topic to be discussed in this chapter is the evaluation of education provided to patients. Whatever means of evaluation are adopted perhaps the most important fact is that some attempt to measure outcome is made. Clearly, the effort involved in patient education can only be justified if it can be shown that there is a tangible benefit to patients. The importance of evaluation in the practice setting was supported by Falvo (1995: 227) who states that: 'Patient education is only as effective as the extent to which it produces measurable outcomes.' But in practice patient teaching is often delivered without any particular form of evaluation.

It is generally acknowledged that in nursing we are not very good at measuring outcomes (French, 1997). Arthur (1995) raises an interesting point associated with the evaluation of educational interventions based on written material. She suggests that despite the widespread use of written patient education material very few studies have been conducted to evaluate the resource:

> Much has been written about readability, but is enough atten-
> tion paid to whether health professionals actually get their
> message across and thereby improve compliance and patient
> satisfaction?

(1085)

Arthur recommends that the costs of producing written information should be balanced against the value accrued from their use. In a clinical situation this would seem to be a valid point. If a great deal of time and effort is to be invested in developing an educational pamphlet then it seems only reasonable that its impact on patients using it should be measured. Measuring impact, however, is a very difficult task and would not usually be associated with practice settings, although it is relevant when conducting research into a newly designed patient education leaflet.

It appears that evaluation is required both in a research context to further develop patient education at a scientific level and also at a practice-based level by individual practitioners to complete the education process. Kiger (1995) also suggests that the benefits to be accrued from planned evaluation of patient teaching are two-fold. First, evaluation can serve to identify both strengths and weaknesses in a teaching approach. If both learners' and teachers' views are taken into account a more rounded perspective can be gained of the process overall. Ultimately, evaluation enables a cost-benefit analysis of a teaching programme to be done. This is an important activity as it is only by demonstrating that teaching can have a demonstrable impact on patient care and quality of life that we can expect it to be adequately resourced. Second, benefits can occur at an individualised level in the context of patient care to provide tangible evidence of what has been accomplished. This, of itself, can serve to motivate patients and staff alike if they can see that they are making progress towards desired outcomes. Evaluation in this chapter is taken to be that concerning direct patient care rather than as part of a research project.

What should be evaluated?

It was mentioned previously that there are three domains of learning, cognitive, psychomotor and affective. The means by which learning outcomes can be evaluated will depend upon the type of learning required of patients. Conventionally we tend to think of the cognitive component of learning: 'What additional information does the person now possess?' However, skills gained or attitudes and perceptions which have been acquired or moderated may also be valuable outcomes of an educational programme. If the goals are relevant to the psychomotor or affective domains then the evaluation must be tailored appropriately to gauge this. Time spent formulating measurable, objective goals will pay dividends at this stage of the process as it will be easier to decide the extent to which they have been achieved. Goals which are vague and have no time frame are very difficult indeed to evaluate.

Evaluation of cognitive learning

Where steps are taken to evaluate learning formally, it can be difficult to decide what exactly should be evaluated and in what way. The most usual way to evaluate patient education is by estimating knowledge gained. The evaluation phase in itself may provide a very important teaching opportunity by encouraging patients to ask their own questions and to address topics which they consider to be particularly important for themselves, so for this reason alone, it should not be left untouched. However, as Wilson-Barnett and Osborne (1983) suggest, it can be difficult to interpret whether the integration of new knowledge is being measured, or simply recall of recently acquired facts, because the time between the teaching intervention and the evaluation is often very short. Whether longer-term retention has been achieved is frequently not reported in research and at a practical level it may not be feasible to gauge the impact of a teaching intervention over time. It will be for nurses working with particular client groups to decide what are the most appropriate short- and long-term goals in terms of disease management and it will be at a one-to-one level with patients that individual goals should be determined.

Evaluation of behavioural change

There is also a school of thought which argues that the measurement of knowledge itself is not always appropriate, since if, for example, behavioural change was the goal of the intervention then it is behaviour which should be evaluated. This would also concur with the definition of patient education adopted for use in this book. To evaluate behavioural change both psychomotor and affective learning will often need to be taken into account. Patients are rarely taught for the sake of knowledge gain alone, but more usually, for the application of the knowledge. Therefore, an evaluation based on knowledge gain may not in itself be particularly valuable. This point can be illustrated with reference to the education of those with diabetes. As Dunn (1988: 503) has remarked:

> The educational model which proposed knowledge improvement as a necessary condition for behaviour change ... is wrong. It ignores the reality that patients fail to comply for many reasons, the least of which is insufficient information.

This perspective is also supported by others, for example, Glasgow and Osteen (1992: 1430). They note that educational programmes are often evaluated according to physiological parameters, such as how much weight has been lost or whether a set of blood results has improved: 'Behaviour not physiology should be the primary . . . outcome for health education.'

However, indicators of behaviour, such as weight change, may be the best means of undertaking evaluation in practice. Moreover, it is not unreasonable to use such proxies, provided it can be demonstrated that they are adequately associated with the desired behaviour.

Falvo (1995: 227) acknowledges the need for both short-term outcomes such as knowledge gain and also the need for a longer-term perspective in which attempts are made to gauge the extent to which knowledge is put into practice. With reference to the needs of those with end-stage renal disease (ESRD) she notes that:

> Specific technical skills, problem solving or coping skills, or self-efficacy may be the most critical mediators of positive outcomes in patient education interventions for ESRD.

How can the outcome be measured?

Evaluating behaviour change can be accomplished if the desired behaviour has been defined and both the patient and the educator understand what and how it is to be measured. This would be, for example, by direct observation, verbal report, completing a diary, or in some cases by physiological indicators of the behaviour.

It was noted earlier in this chapter that the teaching of psychomotor skills was rarely reported. However, one study relevant to this area was conducted to evaluate the way in which elderly people were able to use inhalers as a consequence of a patient teaching programme. The author (Abley, 1997) reports how she developed a checklist of points relevant to inhaler technique. She scored patients both before and after teaching them how to use their device and as a consequence of her study was able to conclude that the teaching did lead to an improvement in inhaler technique. However, she did note that further work was required to investigate whether the improvement could be sustained over time. This is a valuable study because it illustrates how education can be evaluated in a simple practical way.

An important point about measuring outcome is that thought and preparation is required prior to the teaching itself. If changes in knowledge, skills or attitudes are to be measured quantitatively it presupposes that there is some instrument by which this task can be achieved. It may be feasible to use instruments developed and validated by others; alternatively, they will need to be developed at a local level. As there is very little time available for the total activity of patient education it may be assumed that evaluation instruments must be simple and quick to use and suitable from both the nurse's and patient's point of view. Consider the progress which has been made in the measurement of pain in recent years to develop pain thermometers and scales which are readily applicable in a fast-moving clinical environment. Similar developments will be required in other areas of patient care if changes in both pre- and post-education settings are to be measured in a practical way.

For some it is the education process in itself which is of importance, rather than specified outcomes, thus *measuring* outcomes may not be considered valuable. For example, Feste and Anderson (1995), who have worked extensively to facilitate the empowerment of people with diabetes, would argue that many of the traditional parameters used to evaluate teaching programmes are inappropriate:

> The traditional compliance approach to health care views health education as a process that both persuades and prepares patients to carry out recommendations made by health professionals. Its major emphasis is on acquiring the knowledge and skills necessary to carry out a prescribed healthcare regimen. Because of this narrow view of health, the effectiveness of patient education is determined initially by its impact on treatment adherence and, ultimately, by its effect on the physiological endpoints related to health and disease.
>
> (140)

Therefore, if the educational programme has been designed to promote empowerment, evaluation should focus on the extent to which patients have been able to achieve their own goals rather than pre-selected goals of health professionals. These may be identifiable but not measurable, although, in psychotherapy, behaviour therapists have made considerable strides in applying rigorous measurement to client-defined goals (see, for example, Marks *et al.*, 1977; Newell, 1994). However, for people with a chronic illness it has been recommended that patient education should focus on the experiences of the person living with the condition, and that they should be encouraged to reflect on what works well and what they find difficult, to consider the resources available to themselves and then to consider how they may be used to their own advantage. Evaluation then focuses on the extent to which they feel they have made progress. None of this is incompatible with the idea of measurement of outcome, but it is a completely different focus from the examination of biological parameters such as blood results.

What should be done if learning outcomes are not achieved?

It is also possible that if an evaluation indicates poor outcomes it is not necessarily because the patients were not well taught. After a teaching programme, patients may not have made the progress which nurses may have intended. There is a tendency to view this as a failure of the teaching intervention, but it must also be acknowledged that patients have an element of free will and may not wish to change, to adhere to advice, or to learn information that has been offered them. As Ruzicki (1989: 629) has commented, 'nurses must give up their feelings of guilt if their patients don't learn or don't want to learn'.

As Thompson (1984) has pointed out, non-compliance is not restricted to health care situations. The advice of a range of professionals may, or may not, be followed by clients or customers. This is seen as part of human rights: failure to follow advice does not carry with it a judgement about the person. A decision not to follow proffered advice may be seen as a statement of independence. Thompson suggested that if the topic of clients choosing not to accept or follow advice is studied at all by other professionals it is most likely to be 'in terms of necessary improvements in the services they offer' (115). Perhaps it is time for nurses to do likewise. If patients choose not to follow advice it may be that the advice or the services require closer inspection.

However, lack of success in achieving patient education outcomes may be related to inadequate or inappropriate teaching and in such instances the way patient education has been planned and delivered must be carefully considered. In nursing we must acknowledge that there are still many areas of patient education for which we do not have a sufficient knowledge base and such areas require further research. For example, Wilson-Barnett (1997) draws our attention to how inadequately we understand how we should teach patients to cope with pain, yet this is a legitimate area of work in nursing. One area where considerable detailed consideration has been given is that of education for those with arthritis, as illustrated in Figure 5.11.

I   INTRODUCTION

Background

Patient education is a powerful strategy intervention that can improve the lives of persons with rheumatic disease. Most forms of arthritis are chronic in nature and extend over many years. Therefore, along with the routine, ongoing education given by caregivers during individual clinical contacts, the patient needs a formal body of knowledge and skills in order to manage the disease on a day-to-day basis. Effective, efficient management of chronic disease is possible only when patients are knowledgeable participants in decisions about their care and are able to follow through on these decisions.

Patient education is considered an integral part of the treatment of the more than 100 forms of rheumatic disease. More than 75 education programs, reported in the literature, have shown beneficial effects on various aspects of health status, such as functional ability, psychological state, and pain. Furthermore, considerable effort has been made to develop and/or test instruments to evaluate important health outcomes of rheumatic disease care.

This document addresses suggested standards for formal rheumatic disease patient education programs. The purposes of the standards are to: (1) assure the quality of patient education programs, (2) promote the easy access to education for the patient with rheumatic disease, and (3) secure documentation of outcomes of patient education that can be used to improve care.

Definitions

The following terms are defined for use in this document.

1.   **Patient Education**. Patient education is planned, organized learning experiences designed to facilitate voluntary adoption of behaviors or beliefs conducive to health. It is a set of planned educational activities

that are separate from clinical patient care. The activities of a patient education program must be designed to attain goals the patient has participated in formulating. The primary focus of these activities includes acquisition of information, skills, beliefs and attitudes which impact on health status, quality of life, and possibly health care utilization.

2. **Program**. A program consists of three parts:
    a. Specific objectives oriented to each individual or group
    b. Content tailored to meet these objectives
    c. Education processes which deliver the content in a manner which enables the patient to achieve the objectives

    A program can be delivered in a variety of ways and in different settings dependent upon the needs of patients and the availability of resources.

3. **Standards**. Standards are written statements that describe the expectations of the quality of a given education program.

4. **Review Criteria**. Review criteria are measurable methods of determining whether the standards have been met.

5. **Provider**. The provider may be an individual practitioner, an organization or an institution. In all cases the provider is responsible for upholding the standards.

6. **Approved Program**. An approved program is one that has been found to meet the rheumatic disease patient education standards as determined by the designated authority.

II NEEDS ASSESSMENT STANDARDS
Standard

The numbers and needs of persons with rheumatic disease vary. Therefore, patient education programs must begin with an assessment of the needs of the target population. This includes the patient and his/her family members and significant care providers.

The provider of the patient education program will conduct an educational needs assessment of the target patient population. This assessment will include, but not be limited to, problems caused by the rheumatic disease, skills needed to manage the disease, and current level of knowledge and skills. Preferred language of instruction and reading level will also be assessed, if applicable. Additional need assessments, as appropriate, may be conducted with health care providers, administrators, or family members and significant others.

Review Criterion
The provider will document how the needs assessment was conducted and the findings of the needs assessment.

III PLANNING/MANAGEMENT STANDARDS
Standard
Planning is a comprehensive process that should involve health professionals and educators as well as persons with rheumatic diseases and members of their families.

In addition, it entails good communication and clearly delineated responsibilities and functions. Communication must occur among program personnel, health care givers, community health agencies, patients, and their family members. A program coordinator with ultimate responsibility and authority for the quality and operation of the program should be designated. The program should be readily accessible to all patients for whom it has been designed.

Review Criteria
Provider will document the participation of a rheumatologist, one or more other health professionals and patients in the selection or planning of a program.

Each provider will designate one person as coordinator. At a minimum, this person will be responsible for coordinating and documenting patient education activities and is responsible for the quality and operation of the program.

Information about each patient's participation shall be retained in a patient's record or similar file for at least 5 years. This record will be available for the patient's personal or other consented use.

IV CURRICULUM STANDARDS
Standard
The program curriculum organizes the content and documents the educational process. It is also expected that the educational program will be reasonably supported by professional consensus and the research literature on arthritis patient education.

The provider periodically assesses the availability of community sources for their potential contribution to rheumatic disease education. In addition, programs should be updated in a timely manner.

Review Criteria

The program shall have written patient outcome objectives which reflect the findings of the needs assessment(s) and the patients' goals.

The program shall offer information and skills in the content areas determined by the needs assessment and patients' goals. These will be documented by a written curriculum plan which includes content outlines, instructional methods, and instructional materials.

Documentation is available to show that curriculum and instructional materials are appropriate for the specified target audience. The curriculum is reviewed and updated as necessary or at least every 5 years.

The provider shows evidence of an initial assessment of community resources and repeats the assessment at least every 2 years. The assessment includes the name, address, telephone number and a brief statement of what the particular resource offers.

V INSTRUCTOR STANDARDS

Qualified personnel are essential to the success of a rheumatic disease education program. Instructors should have recent training and experience in both rheumatic disease and educational principles, including teaching approaches specific to the target audience (e.g., children, adults, geriatric, culturally diverse population, etc.).

Review Criteria (instructor-led patient education)

1. Instructors are health professionals or lay persons with special education and/or training and experience appropriate to the instructional needs of the program.
2. Documentation of rheumatic disease related training and/or experience is provided.
3. Personnel are expected to participate in continuing education in their areas of expertise on a regular basis.
4. Evidence is provided of regular meetings between instructors and program coordinator.

Review Criteria (mediated patient education)

1. Some educational programs such as those utilizing interactive computers, interactive video, or packages utilizing written, audio tape, and/or video components do not require an instructor. When such programs are used, a person knowledgeable in program content and rheumatology care must be readily available to answer questions or

assist with problems. Access may be in person or by telephone. Resource persons for mediated programs must meet the same criteria as outlined in section V, 1–4.

VI EVALUATION STANDARDS

Standard

In order for a program to meet the standards of this document, it must demonstrate its effectiveness in maintaining or improving health status (i.e., pain, functional ability, psychological state, social functioning, and/or quality of life). For example, decreased pain, depression, disability, fatigue, and improvement of quality of life can be determined by assessing the patient with a standardized measurement tool. Maintenance and/or improvement may be shown in terms of group or individual change (e.g., a third of a standard deviation) or other definitions that can be justified by the provider. In addition, satisfaction data from patients and family members must be collected and reviewed annually.

Review Criteria

For new, not previously approved, programs.

1. Effectiveness is documented by scores on standard validated instruments.
2. Providers do not need to present new evaluation data when using already approved programs.
3. Any provider who chooses to use an approved program which has been demonstrated to meet the criteria in section VI, 1 for patients who differ in some major way from the patient groups for which the program was designed, must show evidence that the program is effective for this new patient group.

Figure 5.11 Arthritis and musculoskeletal patient education standards – an example

An example of patient education standards
– an illustration of good practice

Burckhardt (1994) published standards for the education of patients with arthritis. These standards are a very important milestone because, as Lorig and Visser point out:

1 they define patient education in terms of educational interventions;
2 the standards involve patient input and are focused on patient goals;
3 the standards recognise the ability of both professionals and lay people to become patient educators if they have had sufficient preparation;
4 the standards have very rigorous evaluation criteria.

The standards are included in this chapter as they are a wonderful example of the rigour with which patient education should be undertaken.

Burckhardt (1994) raised the entire profile of patient education by stating that patient education programmes must meet these standards and must be able to demonstrate their value in terms of meeting the stated objectives of the intervention.

How many patient teaching interventions could currently demonstrate this form of impact? Yet why not? It is important that patient education is accepted as an integral part of care but this goal will only be achieved if the time and energy invested in it can be shown to improve patients' quality of life in some way. According to Lorig and Visser (1994):

> By demanding that our interventions be judged in terms of patient outcomes, we move the role of such education from that of nice but unnecessary adjunct to medical treatment to a necessary part of standard medical care. ... This criterion moves patient education into the realm of treatment by insisting that the program be demonstrated to be effective on health status.
>
> (4)

Conclusion

The challenges imposed by the current health care climate are acknowledged, but patients' needs for education are undiminished. Nurses are therefore in a difficult situation in which there is evidence that their clients require patient education to be provided but the time in which teaching can occur is very limited. Research-based information about teaching interventions and evaluation of education has been reviewed. From this material there will be some studies which readers will find potentially applicable to their own areas of work and in this way can help to enhance evidence-based practice. The chapter is completed with the inclusion of patient education standards which serve as exemplars of good practice.

KEY POINTS FROM CHAPTER 5

1 *Building on the work of Chapter 4*, this chapter is concerned with intervention and evaluation of patient education.

2 *Teaching based on verbal interventions is the most commonly used form of patient education but frequently is not done well.* Points to bear in mind include allowing enough time to deliver the required amount of information, delivering it at an appropriate time, providing a consistent message and clarifying how patients may receive ongoing information.

3 *Verbal teaching requires that nurses must possess appropriate communication skills* in addition to having appropriate knowledge of the topic to be taught.

4 *Written material is a useful adjunct to verbal teaching* and is widely used. However, for written educational material to be successful careful preparation is required. Research reveals that a substantial amount of existing patient education requires reading abilities above the level of the majority of patients.

5 *The readability of the material:* size of print, use of space, colour and cartoons, type of paper and the cultural background of consumers will all have an impact on the success of written patient educational material.

6 *Audio and audio-visual teaching material* can be used with success but should be considered as a means of supplementing face-to-face contact rather than as a replacement for it.

7 *Computer-based teaching interventions* are rapidly being developed and while they are not widely used at present are likely to be used increasingly as access to hardware and software sophistication increases.

8 *Teaching patients psychomotor skills* is an important educational activity which accounts for a substantial amount of nursing time. However, the evidence upon which to base principles of this aspect of patient education is extremely sparse.

9 *Planned, structured teaching involving reinforcement and more than one strategy* offers the best chance of successful teaching, whilst unplanned, *ad hoc* teaching on an opportunist basis is not recommended.

10 *Evaluation is a crucial stage in the education process* but is often overlooked. Evaluation is required both to further our understanding of successful teaching interventions and also to enable patients to appreciate the extent of any progress they make towards achieving desired goals.

11 *Selection of outcome measures and methods* will depend upon the objectives of the education and the need to take account of cognitive, psychomotor and affective learning.

12 *Patient education standards* developed to enhance education for those with arthritis are presented as an example of good practice.

Chapter 6

Educational issues relating to people with long-term health problems

Introduction

Building on the work of the previous two chapters, we will now turn to a concentration on specific issues which must be taken into account when aiming to help individuals undertake self-management programmes for chronic health problems.

This chapter will begin by reconsidering the definition of patient education which was discussed in Chapter 1 and which is used to focus our thoughts on the subject throughout this book. From this definition we see that the goal of patient education is often behavioural. For patients with a chronic rather than an acute condition, the behavioural change must be sustained for long periods of time, possibly for life. Indeed, sustaining such changes in behaviour may well have extremely important consequences for the patient's continued well-being. By contrast, failure to carry on with long-term behaviour change may significantly impair the person's functioning, or even be life-threatening, in just the same way as problems with absorbing information in acute settings. As a result, the need for excellent teaching approaches is just as great in the case of long-term health problems as in acute care. Indeed, because of the necessity for the client to carry out behavioural change over a long period of time, usually without supervision, the skill of the nurse in teaching and, importantly, motivating the patient, may face a greater challenge than in these acute settings.

The majority of patients and clients live in the community rather than a hospital and so must manage an illness or health problem without much supervision. Research illustrates that many patients are often unable to sustain self-management regimens and healthy behaviour, and the implications of this for patient education will be discussed. Issues which influence educational interventions aiming to enable people to manage chronic health problems in a primary care setting will be explored.

Definition of patient education

The working definition of patient education adopted for this book is:

> planned combinations of learning activities designed to assist people who are having or have had experience with illness or disease in making changes in their behaviour conducive to health.
>
> (Squyres 1980: 1, adapted from Green *et al.*, 1979)

In nursing we have often considered patient education as a short-term intervention which is principally to help patients gain knowledge and skills. In some patient situations this is essential and it is sufficient. For example, in pre-operative care, patients may require knowledge to understand what will happen to them whilst in hospital and to perform pre-operative breathing and leg exercises. Once they have successfully recovered from their operations, patients may no longer need the information and they don't need to continue to do the breathing exercises. However, as we noted in Chapter 1, the majority of patients receiving health care at present have chronic health problems. Indeed a recent prediction for North America indicated that about 70 per cent of health care will be in a primary care setting in the next decade and thus only 30 per cent will be given in secondary and tertiary settings (Zungalo, 1997), a reversal of the conventional concept of care giving. A similar situation can be expected in the United Kingdom by the year 2010 (D.o.H., 1994).

The implications of this great change in the organisation of nursing care will be felt both in professional education and practice (Clark, 1997), and the need for better educational and motivational skills may be one of the most major aspects of change. Patients with chronic health problems may need to retain knowledge and skills for many years. For example, patients with hypertension, arthritis, diabetes, cancer, or mental health problems may have no speedy relief from their health problems and, in consequence, will need to self-manage them for a prolonged period, possibly for life. Yet research indicates that many people do not self-manage health problems for sustained amounts of time.

Four crucially important questions are:

1. Why do people change their behaviour?
2. How do people change and learn to change?
3. How can nurses and the health care team stimulate learning and change?
4. How can patient education be integrated into their treatment?

(adapted from Gruninger, 1995: 16)

During the course of this chapter and the next, issues relating to these questions will be explored, but unfortunately, few clear-cut answers emerge.

Self-management of chronic health problems

From a traditional health professional perspective the management of chronic illness is a simple issue: health is everyone's priority, so people will follow the treatment regimen to promote their health. Unfortunately, there is plenty of research evidence to indicate that management regimens are not followed (Wainwright and Gould, 1997; Cramer and Spilker, 1991; Cameron and Gregor, 1987; Roth, 1987; DiMatteo and DiNicola, 1982).

The issue of compliance has been reported to affect a wide range of health care behaviours, conditions and age groups including after organ transplant (Wainwright and Gould, 1997); kidney transplant (Rovelli *et al.*, 1989); hormone replacement (Rozenberg *et al.*, 1995); asthma (Bosley *et al.*, 1995); mental illness (Engstrom, 1991); amongst children (Rapoff and Barnard, 1981); amongst adolescents (Kyngas and Hentinen, 1995); and with the elderly (Owens *et al.*, 1991; Working Party of the Royal College of Physicians, 1984). Are patients who do not follow health care regimens foolish, wilful, uncooperative? This seems unlikely, particularly given the dire consequences which so often result from non-adherence to medical and nursing instructions regarding chronic ill-health and its management. A major part of the solution may be educational, but the picture is complex and the best form of educational programme is not fully understood. None the less, non-compliance is considered to be a very serious health care problem which urgently needs to be addressed (Jones *et al.*, 1991).

The troublesome concept of compliance

Maintaining behavioural change to manage or treat a health problem has often been referred to as compliance and patients who do not sustain behavioural change are said to be non-compliant. Compliance has been simply defined as: 'following the instructions of the health care provider' (Cramer, 1991: 3).

Cameron (1996), citing Davis (1968) suggests that compliance can be both an attitude and a behaviour:

> Compliance as an attitude is willingness or intention to follow health prescription. Compliance as a behaviour is related to the actual carrying out of prescriptions.
>
> (245)

Compliance and non-compliance are considered by some to be value-laden terms implying a negative judgement upon the patient (DiMatteo and DiNicola, 1982; Simons 1992). The concept of compliance implies that patients passively do what they are told to do by health professionals. It has even been suggested that 'the word compliance is repugnant to many educators because it implies sub-servience, dependence, and unquestioning obedience to authority' (D'Onofrio, 1980: 271).

Of course, these are just the opposite qualities and behaviours from those which many health professionals are trying to achieve in their clients. Whether the prescribed action is that patients take medication of the right amount at the right times, exercise more, reduce their salt intake or reduce activities that cause them to feel stressed, they all require that the patient has the information in the first place. Thus all patient education requires the giving of information. However, to achieve any of these actions requires the patient to *apply* their knowledge and it is at this stage that literature indicates that patients may be unable to change behaviour in order to promote their health. Thus, following advice is not a passive event. Putting knowledge into practice is an activity which involves many variables.

Other phrases such as adherence (Jenkins, 1995) or self-care behaviour (Shillitoe and Christie, 1990) have been recommended. For want of an alternative but succinct term, compliance will be used here to describe the maintenance of health behaviour but its limitations are fully accepted. Thorne (1990) coins the phrase 'constructive noncompliance' to address the situation in which patients decide against following a prescribed regimen, not as 'an irrational response complicating a pre-existing medical condition' (67) but rather as a carefully thought through decision-making process in which they find that a change from the prescribed strategy may be in their best long-term interests. So to say that patients are either 'compliant' or 'non-compliant' is an oversimplification.

As following prescribed treatment regimens and enabling people to self-manage chronic health problems often form a substantial part of the goals of patient education, this issue is seen as being highly relevant to the topic of patient and client education. Unfortunately we do not yet know which factors are most influential in patient self-management. What we do know is that the situation is complex, dynamic and that the same factors will not apply to each person, condition or illness.

The relationship between knowledge and behaviour

The complexity of the relationship between knowledge and behaviour will be illustrated with reference to previous work undertaken by Coates (1993) and Coates and Boore (1996). Patient education is a fundamental aspect of care for people with diabetes to help them to control the disease, remain symptom free, to prevent or delay the onset of acute or chronic complications and to help promote a good quality of life. It may be assumed that increased knowledge about self-management should foster good control of diabetes but it is a rather controversial point with some findings suggesting knowledge has a positive effect upon diabetes control (Brown, 1990) whilst other research (Dunn et al., 1990) suggests that level of knowledge will not predict improved control. The study by Coates (1993) aimed, first, to assess the respondents' knowledge of diabetes and its management and second, to assess whether knowledge of diabetes was related to diabetes control. The study was of a survey design comprising three phases. In the first knowledge and beliefs about health were assessed via a postal questionnaire sent to all adults aged between 18 and 35 years who were registered at one of two large general hospital diabetic outpatient clinics. The second stage involved the gathering of clinical details from patients' notes and the third comprised semi-structured interviews with a sub-sample of twenty people.

Knowledge was assessed by means of a structured questionnaire and metabolic control was evaluated by an index of long-term blood glucose referred to as glycosylated haemoglobin. The questionnaire, which had been designed by Dunn *et al.* (1984) was returned by 275 adults aged between 18 and 35 years.

The mean knowledge result was found to be very good, with patients having a mean score of 16.6 out of a possible total of 19, implying that the people in the sample were knowledgeable about the principles of self-management. Yet the mean glycosylated haemoglobin result of 10.1 per cent was approximately a third greater than the figure of 7.4 per cent said to represent the upper limit of the normal non-diabetic range. Although these people were knowledgeable, their diabetic control was not as good as it would need to be to prevent long-term diabetic complications. The interview data gathered in the second part of the study indicated that knowledge is only one of several variables which influence metabolic control. The qualitative data indicated lifestyle and beliefs can have a huge impact on behaviour even amongst knowledgeable people as is the case with these individuals. These results support a conclusion drawn by Dunn (1988) and are endorsed by the work of others (Goodall and Halford, 1991).

The conclusion drawn is not one of condemnation of educational programmes. On the contrary, the prerequisites for self-management must be knowledge and skills, but it is emphasised that many variables may influence behaviour. This study offers empirical support for what many good educators may do 'instinctively' – tailor the needs for the educational approach to the individual learner. Since not *all* those involved in education have this instinctive grasp, however, it will be important that careful assessment for teaching, as described in Chapter 4, includes an examination of the personal variables found in this study to effect use of information. Patient education programmes are vital, but the nature of the programme needs to be inclusive of psychological and social influences as well as knowledge and skills. Nurses involved in the education of those with long-term health problems must take a broad view of education when planning teaching programmes. Unfortunately, which variables apply to which individuals is still hotly debated, but some of the themes which are emerging from the literature will be presented below.

Achieving behavioural change

The regimen itself

As the inability to follow prescribed treatment for prolonged periods of time has been such a huge problem in health care it has received considerable attention, in order to understand factors which may predict those who are likely or unlikely to follow health care regimens. If the principal factors in this issue were known they could be taken into account when planning patient education. Strauss and Glaser (1975) conducted pioneering work into understanding problems associated with managing long-term health problems: 'At first blush, regimen management may not seem a problem of much magnitude: regimens are either followed by obedient, sensible patients or ignored at their peril' (21).

In order to follow any programme, patients must first know what to do, and so knowledge must play a part in the long-term management of health problems. Once the person has understood that they must undertake some form of health care regimen the next vital step is that they learn what is involved in it. As Strauss and Glaser (1975) point out, regimens have specific characteristics: they may involve excluding something such as some food in a diet or particular types of sport or exertion, they may entail adding something such as medicines or exercises. Some procedures can be quite complicated, such as if a person has a Hickman line which needs flushing each day or has to learn to dialyse at home. Some of the regimens to be followed may also create considerable anxiety: 'At the initial session of learning how to give insulin shots, the mother of a diabetic child shook so much that she dropped the needle and burst into tears' (Benoliel cited by Strauss and Glaser, 1975: 22).

Once patients know what to do there are many factors which influence whether information will be put into practice. Strauss and Glaser (27) suggest the questions listed in Figure 6.1 should be answered by health professionals relating to the regimen itself when teaching patients in order to appreciate some of the factors which may influence ability to maintain a health care regimen.

If there are negative responses to one or more of these questions it is easy to imagine why even a person who is knowledgeable about a health care regimen may find it difficult to put the information into practice. For example, a woman of 49 years was prescribed high doses of steroids to help treat pulmonary hypertension. The

---

1   Is it difficult or easy to learn and to carry out?

2   Does it take much time?

3   Does it cause much discomfort or pain?

4   Does it cause side effects, especially if they are actually or apparently risky ones?

5   Does it need much effort or energy to carry out?

6   Is it visible to others?

7   If known, might it cause others to stigmatise the person?

8   Does it seem efficient?

9   Is it expensive?

10   Does it lead to increasing social isolation?

Figure 6.1   Questions to be answered about the nature of a health care regimen

steroids were leading to weight gain, water retention and hirsutism. This led to a reluctance to be seen outside and thus contributed to social isolation. Whilst on the steroids she was not feeling any better, indeed some days she felt worse than before she started treatment. These factors then mitigated against her taking the steroids even though she was aware that they were part of her recommended treatment and her condition was potentially life-threatening.

Wainwright and Gould (1997) also mention some of these issues in relation to non-adherence with medications in organ transplant patients. They note that the toxic side-effects of immunosuppressants such as cyclosporin had led to some people omitting some of their tablets, to the extent that, citing the work of Didlake *et al.* (1988), some patients rejected their transplanted kidney – a high price to pay for 'non-adherence'. This problem relates to the third and fourth of Strauss and Glaser's questions, indicating that they are pertinent and in the long term cannot be ignored. Patients must be made fully aware of the potential consequences of their actions and, preferably, less toxic treatment regimens are required. Indeed, the pharmaceutical companies are currently developing immunosuppressants which have less disabling side-effects while remaining efficient therapeutic agents.

Although the work of Strauss and Glaser (1975) was published over twenty years ago, it therefore still appears to be relevant to the clinical situations facing patients today. They stress the important fact that patients' chronic illnesses and their associated regimens are secondary to daily living. Most people do not want their lifestyle to be seriously affected in order to manage their health. Thus if a prescribed health care routine presents more difficulties than the symptoms themselves patients may have little inclination to follow the regimen. Health care professionals must accept that regimens are not automatically accepted. Indeed, they are often judged on a social rather than a medical basis. Such a perspective would be supported by others, for example, Becker and Rosenstock (1984) and Cameron and Gregor (1987), who acknowledge that the perspectives of health professionals and patients and clients can be quite different.

Graveley and Oseasohn (1991) investigated the issue of people who do not take prescribed medication. Their study involved 249 men over 64 years of age who were prescribed from one to seven tablets daily. Compliance was judged according to a pill count undertaken on two home visits. They found that 73 per cent of the sample were non-compliant. The method of pill counting has its limitations (Gordis, 1976; Rosenvinge et al., 1990) but all ways of determining compliance have some associated problems. In an attempt to identify factors which would lead to non-compliant behaviour a range of variables were studied, including age, marital status, living alone, locus of control and depression. Ethnicity and number of tablets to be taken daily were the only ones found to have a significant effect. The greater the number of pills a person had to take the more likely they were to be non-compliant. Ethnicity, in this study, refers to people being 'Anglo' (54 per cent) or 'non-Anglo' (46 per cent) comprising Hispanic, Black and Asian. Anglos were reported to be significantly more compliant than non-Anglos. However, the mean number of years of education was greater for Anglos than for non-Anglos, thus it may be this rather than ethnicity itself that is most important. The sample members were also interviewed and report many reasons why tablets had not been taken, such as not re-ordering a repeat prescription in time, difficulties associated with taking tablets prescribed 6-hourly, breaking tablets to take a half tablet, not being aware that a dose had been altered and 'taking TID with meal medication when they only ate two meals a day' (Graveley and Oseasohn, 1991: 57). These qualitative results suggest that patients must be consulted when regimens are drawn up. This would appear to be a logical step and would concur with the philosophy proposed by Szasz and Hollender (1956) which was discussed in Chapter 1.

Psycho-social issues

Cultural differences which may influence educational interventions were investigated by Wierenga and Wuethrich (1995) and support the previously cited study in that they found there were differences between Caucasian and African Americans which should be taken into account when planning an educational programme. As a result of their study they recommend that, although there were socio-economic differences between the two cultural groups in their study, these should not be assumed. Rather they emphasise the need for careful, individualised assessment of clients to check aspects of self-management which they feel they could cope with and those they could not. The emphasis of an educational intervention may need to vary according to the assessment results. This is an important point because in nursing we often have a concept of a standard package of information required for patients with diagnosed diseases, rather than thinking about the person first and the medical condition second. Such standard packages go some way towards addressing information needs, but do not tackle either personal variations in need for information or how to make the information optimally reinforcing for the patient.

Bosley *et al.* (1995) investigated reasons for non-compliance with asthma therapy: 102 patients with asthma aged 18–70 years who were prescribed regular inhaled corticosteroids and beta-agonists were involved in the study. Of the 72 people who completed the study, 37 'took less than 70 per cent of the prescribed dose over the study period or omitted doses for 1 week and were defined as non-compliant' (899). The study is reported to indicate that non-compliance 'is associated with a complex mix of psycho-social factors'. However, no factor had a significant relationship with compliance behaviour. No significant difference between age, duration of condition, sex or socioeconomic status was identified. Further investigation into these psycho-social factors and the possible usefulness of psychological intervention to improve compliance is recommended.

Studies such as those of Graveley and Oseasohn (1991), Wierenga and Wuethrich (1995) or Bosley *et al.* (1995) are typical of much of the work in this area, in that no single study seems able to indicate the vital variables to be addressed to understand compliance. Leventhal and Cameron (1987) also comment on the great variability in results:

> This variability suggests that non-compliance is a multi-factor problem that is influenced by the characteristics of the disease, the treatment regimen and setting, as well as a variety of both relatively stable dispositions and highly variable states of the participant.
>
> (118)

Cameron (1996) comments on this issue and notes that problems with research in this area include that definitions of 'compliance' vary as do the parameters which lead a person to be labelled as either 'compliant' or 'non-compliant'; measurement of the concept is variable. Not surprisingly the results of studies also differ and some contradict. It is perhaps only when a large volume of literature is reviewed and appraised that trends may emerge. For example, Cameron identified over 200 factors which have been studied to find those linked to compliance behaviour. She organised them into the following five broad groups:-

1   Knowledge and understanding (includes communication)
2   Quality of interaction
3   Social isolation and social support
4   Health beliefs and attitudes
5   Illness and treatment

Through analysing the vast range of work on this subject Cameron (1996) believes that there is enough evidence available to guide health professionals involved in patient teaching to help ensure that the most effective teaching programmes are designed. She recommends that health professionals involved in patient education should take these categories into account as follows:

> The patient should be given information which is clear and unambiguous and their understanding should be assessed. A sensitive empathetic approach by the practitioner is important

and he/she should be knowledgeable about the factors influencing compliance, and should try to understand the patients' motives, demands and expectations as well as their health beliefs.

(248)

It is interesting to note that demographic factors, personality characteristics, level of knowledge and social norms or patient characteristics have not been consistently identified as causing non-compliance. According to Cramer: 'Compliance can be total, partial, nil or erratic. Neither age, education, nor socio-economic level makes a difference in how patients use therapeutic plans' (Cramer, 1991: 4).

Theoretical models to help explain or predict health behaviour

The information presented above illustrates that a simple linear relationship between knowledge and behaviour is inadequate and that a more complex approach to patient education is required. Leventhal and Cameron (1987) suggest that trying to advance our understanding on a trial and error basis is unlikely to be successful, rather that: 'Theoretical analysis of the compliance problem is essential for forward movement' (118) may be needed to assist us. Many theories and models have been proposed to help explain or predict health behaviour. Several of the more commonly known models are briefly outlined below.

Biomedical model

This model is based on the traditional approach to medical care in Western society. Disease is of a biological origin and treatment and management of health problems are based on biological theories. In this model variables such as age, patient income, education, severity of disease and complexity of regimen are thought to affect self-management behaviour. Variables such as age or severity of disease are not amenable to modification, whatever the educational intervention, but greater understanding of their influence may help promote good practice. Other variables in this category are amenable to influence, such as if the treatment regimen was too complicated steps could be taken to simplify it. This model is perhaps the most familiar in many patient education contexts and is described further in Kiger (1995).

As Leventhal and Cameron (1987) point out, because social and psychological characteristics have not been consistently identified as causing non-compliance, this may lend support to the view that a biomedical model is as useful as any other. However, other work (Engel, 1977; Allen and Hall, 1988) has clearly indicated that in this century health and illness cannot be adequately explained by a purely biomedical model. It is likely that the passive patient approach will be fostered by a biomedical approach to patient teaching, so is not too suitable in situations where patient participation and self-management skills are to be encouraged. This issue was discussed in Chapter 1.

Behavioural/social learning

These models draw from theorists such as Pavlov and Skinner (outlined by Ogier, 1989) and are based on the premise that compliance is a behaviour, thus behaviour must be changed if a new regimen or protocol is to be followed. The model involves cues and rewards. Fisher (1992) reports that it has been found to work better on long- rather than short-term treatments, for example stopping smoking or losing weight. This approach is critiqued by Leventhal and Cameron (1987) who quite rightly point out that while promoting an automatic response to cues, these models do not allow for the cognitive processes that will influence behaviour. Thus personal choice, attitudes and emotions do not seem to feature in these approaches to learning. However, later learning theory-based approaches recognise the learner as a being who interacts and influences the environment, rather than being passively reinforced by it (e.g. Bandura, 1977).

Communication-based models

Communicating a message from one person to another involves more than just the actual spoken or written component of the message. As Konrad Lorenz, cited by Gruninger (1995: 19) has rather elegantly expressed it:

> What is said is not always heard
> What is heard is not always understood
> What is understood is not always accepted

What is accepted is not always implemented
What is implemented is not always sustained.

In this section some of the factors influencing communication as an educational medium will be explored.

According to Leventhal and Cameron (1987) communication models are based upon the following six steps:

1 message is sent
2 message is received
3 patient comprehends the message
4 message is retained by the patient
5 message is accepted or believed
6 patient complies

They suggest that the communication model also relatively disempowers patients and clients, who are seen as novices seeking the expert advice of the health educators. However, in long-term illness, such a situation is unlikely to be true as the patients are often the experts in the management of their own condition.

Phillip Ley has undertaken a considerable amount of research into communication in patient education and argues that if patients understand and remember the information given to them they will be better able to comply with the treatment regimens. This approach seems eminently plausible although the research presented by Coates (1993) also suggests that high levels of recalled information may not on their own be sufficient reason to conform to treatment. The model proposed by Ley (1982) is illustrated in Figure 6.2.

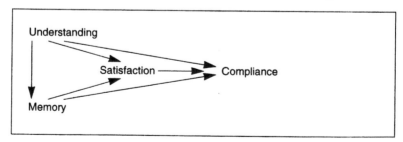

Figure 6.2 A model of the relationships between understanding, memory, satisfaction and compliance

Source: From P. Ley, 'Giving Information to Patients', in R. Eiser, *Social Psychology and Behavioural Science*, © 1982. Reproduced by permission of John Wiley & Sons Limited.

Ley focuses his work on developing strategies to help improve understanding, memory and patients' satisfaction with the information given to them and testing these approaches through research-based inquiry. For example, he advocates making written material easier to read, using illustration to back up written information, and use of humour or cartoons. At the end of his review of research he summarises the situation as follows:

1   patients do not seem to receive as much information as they desire or as professionals judge as adequate;
2   the information provided to patients is often not understood by them, and patients frequently forget what they are told;
3   provision of further information does not lead to adverse consequences;
4   it is possible to improve communications, often with beneficial effects on compliance and recovery.

(Ley, 1982: 365)

Although this work is now quite old, these statements are still applicable today. Further discussion of this model is available in Rutter *et al.* (1993).

Others have also used improved communication as the foundation of their teaching initiative although not necessarily based on Ley's model. Bartlett *et al.* (1984) investigated the effect that interpersonal communication skills and teaching had upon compliance, recall of information and satisfaction with care. They found that the quality of interaction was more important than quantity of information:

Medication adherence was influenced by patient satisfaction with the visit and recall of the regimen, which in turn were determined by the quality of the physician's interpersonal skills and by the amount of patient teaching.

(762)

A much more complicated communication model than Ley's has been proposed by Frederikson (1993).

This model was developed particularly with a view to maximising the communication process between patient and doctor during a medical consultation. The consultation is viewed as an information flow and exchange process. Both patient and doctor begin at the input stage each with their own sets of information, motivation, goals and expectations of the encounter. The process of information exchange then takes place involving verbal exchange, questioning and physical examination of the patient until it is possible for the doctor to formulate a diagnosis and a plan of treatment. It is postulated that what occurs during this stage governs the outcomes of the consultation in terms of perceived satisfaction of both the doctor and the patient. The model by Fredrikson is illustrated in Figure 6.3. This type of careful examination at a conceptual level of an event which is usually taken for granted is an important step in clarifying how information exchange actually occurs. If such a conceptual model is found to work in practice, the deeper understanding of what is happening during a consultation then offers an opportunity to maximise information exchange and hopefully the sense of satisfaction felt by both parties.

This model was used as the framework by which to examine the exchange of information in medical consultations involving a convenience sample of 35 general practitioners (Frederikson, 1995). Following the study it was concluded that: 'attending to the concepts, perception and views of the patient offers a more effective strategy for communication management than a focus on providing

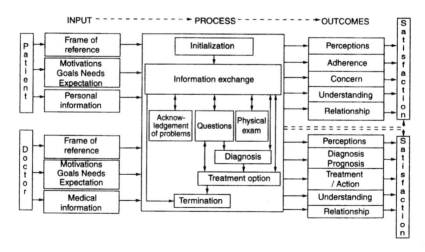

Figure 6.3   Information-exchange model

Source: Reprinted from L.G. Frederikson (1995) 'Exploring information-exchange in consultation: the patient's view of performance and outcomes', *Patients Education Counseling*, 25: 237–46.

vast amounts of standardised information' (Frederikson, 1995, 237). Although this communication model is valuable in that it attempts to clarify what is required in an ideal consultation between a doctor and a patient it contains many variables and thus is conceptually rather difficult to work with.

The importance of communication between doctors and patients was also investigated by Speedling and Rose (1985) who suggest that by increasing patient involvement in the decision-making process patients are more likely to take an active role in disease management. They propose that although the initial interactions may take longer and therefore cost more, if the goals of therapy are to be achieved this approach may save money in the long term.

When critiquing communication approaches Leventhal and Cameron (1987) cite the major deficiency as the lack of explanation about how the information, once received, can lead to attitude and behavioural changes. They do not appear to influence motivation to act. Such an analysis would support the work of Hilton *et al.* (1986). They investigated the education of patients with asthma and reported that both communication issues and psychological factors must be taken into account:

> Good communication skills, listening to the patient's needs and tailoring treatments to each individual is good clinical practice . . . that psychological factors are important in the management of asthma and that psychological interventions may be helpful for some patients who are non-compliant.
>
> (904)

Models which aim to address psychological factors such as attitudes and beliefs which may impinge on behavioural change will be outlined below.

Cognitive approaches

As the nature of disease and health problems has shifted over the last century, so also have the types of models used to explain and understand health and illness. Whilst the medical model still has an important place other models have developed in response to the changing nature of health problems. Cognitive models of behaviour have increasingly been cited in literature relating to health care issues. They are based on the premise that beliefs and attitudes influence the way individuals perceive situations and this affects their behaviour. Two of the models which predominate in the literature, the Health Belief Model (Rosenstock, 1974) and the Theory of Reasoned Action (Fishbein and Ajzen, 1975) are outlined here.

The Health Belief Model was developed by Rosenstock and colleagues initially with reference to health promotion behaviour, but has subsequently been widely applied to the management of chronic illness situations. According to Rosenstock (1974: 2): 'it is the world of the perceiver that determines what he will do and not the physical environment, except as the physical environment comes to be represented in the mind of the behaving individual'.

Thus the Health Belief Model is based on psychological rather than social variables. The principal components of the model are:

1   perceived susceptibility: a person's own view of their health risks which may arise from their condition;
2   perceived severity: a person's own evaluation of the consequences (health and social) of contracting the disease or its side effects.
3   perceived benefits: the benefits the person believes can be gained by following recommended advice;
4   perceived barriers: the negative aspects associated with undertaking recommended health care.

Behaviour is said to be the result of consciously evaluating the above factors. In addition it is suggested that this process is triggered by some cue to action, such as symptoms or a clinic appointment. The Health Belief Model as graphically illustrated by Becker and Maiman (1975) is illustrated in Figure 6.4.

The presumed empirical value of the model is that the beliefs are potentially modifiable. Thus knowledge of relevant attitudes and beliefs would enable educators to take beliefs into account and aim to modify them in order to achieve improved compliance. However, this presumption remains to be justified. A great many teaching programmes based on the Health Belief Model have been developed (Brownlee-Duffeck et al., 1987). A detailed review of the model, based on 48 patient education studies, was published by Janz and Becker (1984) who report that the Health Belief Model is, overall, a valuable framework for explaining health behaviour but later reviews have not been so supportive of the model (Leventhal and Cameron, 1987). According to Rutter et al. (1993) the leading

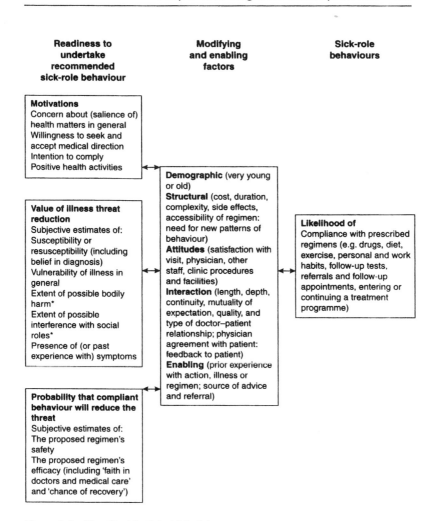

Figure 6.4   The Health Belief Model

Source: From M.H. Becker and L.A. Maiman, 'The Health Belief Model', *Medical Care*, 1975, 13(I): 10–24.

predictor of behaviour is perceived barriers, thus if people do not envisage too many obstacles in fulfilling prescribed health regimens they are more likely to undertake them than those who do. The weakest predictor is that of perceived severity because people find it difficult to imagine severe problems and tend not to be threatened by long-term negative outcomes.

The Theory of Reasoned Action by Fishbein and Ajzen (1975) refers to general beliefs; it is not concerned specifically with health. It is based on the assumption that behaviour is under voluntary control based on a person's beliefs and attitudes towards performing the behaviour and their understanding of the beliefs and attitudes of their significant others regarding the proposed behaviour. Thus information the individual may have about self-management of their health is modified by both their own beliefs and those around them. The model is illustrated in Figure 6.5.

The model is limited in that it assumes that all behaviour is under each individual's control, but in reality some actions may be beyond our control, for example, if we cannot make a clinic appointment due to not having transport (Rutter *et al.*, 1993). The model was subsequently extended to allow for the extent to which individuals believe they can exert control over the behaviour in question. The modified model is referred to as the Theory of Planned Behaviour (Ajzen, 1988).

Reviews of studies based on these models to give further information can be found in Rutter *et al.* (1993), Conner and Norman (1996) and Broome and Llewelyn (1995).

According to Leventhal and Cameron (1987: 126):

> The health belief model and other rational belief models do not deal specifically with coping skills, except to consider the perceived lack of skills as a 'barrier' or 'cost'. Moreover, because of their emphasis on perception and rationality, these models focus exclusively on conscious, intentional behaviour and ignore the wide range of automatic activities that make up so much of daily activity.

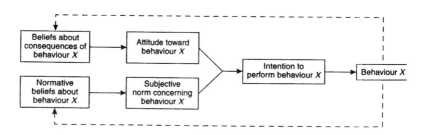

Figure 6.5 The Theory of Reasoned Action

Source: M. Fishbein/I. Ajzen, *Fishbein Belief Attitude Behaviour* (figure 1.2 from page 16). © 1975 Addison Wesley Longman Inc. Reprinted by permission of Addison Wesley Longman.

Although these models and ideas have only been outlined, they serve to illustrate that there is a large volume of research being developed across a number of disciplines, which seeks to clarify our understanding of behavioural change at a theoretical level. No single model has gained acceptance, and probably there will never be any single solution to understanding self-management behaviour.

The Stages of Change Model

A model which helps to explain the process of changing health behaviour rather than the psychological factors underlying it has been developed by Prochaska and DiClemente (1984) and is referred to as The Stages of Change Model. It was developed with a health promotion context in mind; however, it seems applicable to the management of chronic illness. If considered in relation to education it has a valuable contribution because it illustrates that one educational input is unlikely to result in behavioural change; instead, change will occur as a series of steps rather than as a single move. Their model has been portrayed as a circle (Naidoo and Wills, 1994) and as a spiral (Prochaska *et al.*, 1992). Either way, it contains the steps listed in Figure 6.6.

According to Prochaska and DiClemente's model, illustrated in Figure 6.7, simply giving someone information about their condition and how they need to manage should not be expected necessarily to bring about change in behaviour; in itself, it may not be enough to lead to change. If this can be acknowledged, leading to a realisation that education and support must be ongoing, it may enable educators to have greater acceptance of relapses which can be expected and then worked on to help them to be overcome. Basler (1995) examined the issue of changing behaviour and supports the use of Prochaska and DiClemente's model. He points out that it helps us move away from the bi-polar view of health being either good or bad, as though there were a dramatic change from one stable state to another, i.e. from unhealthy to healthy behaviour.

The work of Wall *et al.* (1995), who investigated adherence to Zidovudine (AZT) amongst those with HIV infection, would also support this approach. They found that daily supervised contact helped improve compliance but only whilst the programme lasted. When the supervision declined so did adherence. A model such as

Precontemplation:	the person is not considering changing behaviour at all.
Contemplation:	the person is aware that a change in behaviour is advisable but is not yet ready to do so.
Preparing to change:	the person decides that the potential benefits of changing behaviour could outweigh the barriers (attitudinal, financial, social or personal) they would have to overcome but the individual is not yet ready to change.
Making the change:	the person changes behaviour, in this context in order to self-manage their condition; at this stage they need support and reinforcement.
Maintenance:	the person is able to sustain their behavioural changes.

Figure 6.6   Steps in the Stages of Change Model

that of Prochaska and DiClemente helps alert patient educators to the fact that ongoing supervision is to be expected if desired behaviour is to be sustained.

Many other frameworks and models by which to explain health behaviour have been developed, for example that of Folkman and Lazarus (1985) concerning behaviour to cope with stress, Leventhal *et al.*'s (1984) self-regulatory model of illness behaviour, or Bandura's (1977) social learning theory relating to changing behaviour in order to cope with stress.

The theoretical model deemed most suitable by an educator will be influenced according to professional background and client group. Although no attempt is made to include all potential models it is argued that it is important for educators to consider the premise upon which they base their teaching.

For example, Fisher (1992) evaluated five theoretical models proposed by Leventhal and Cameron (1987) for their suitability as the basis for patient education from a pharmacist's perspective. The models were: biomedical, behavioural/social learning, communication, rational beliefs and self-regulation systems.

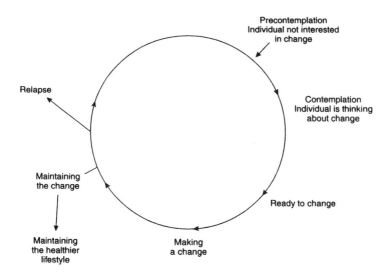

Figure 6.7   The Stages of Change Model (Prochaska and DiClemente, 1984)

Source: Reprinted from J. Naidoo and J. Wills, *Health Promotion: Foundations for Practice*, © 1994, by permission of the publisher WB Saunders Company Limited, London.

Fisher's preferred approach to patient education after appraising each one was the communication model, although according to the information presented above the impact of this strategy alone would need to be critically evaluated. However, the importance of Fisher's article is that he has identified that practice must be theoretically driven. He critically reviewed a range of theoretical approaches, selected the one he considered to be the most applicable to his profession and then recommended how pharmacists could improve their patient education based on the communication model:

> Pharmacists that utilize positive, comprehensive communication skills can better educate patients. . . . For pharmacists to take an active role in patient education, it is imperative that they develop the necessary communication skills. . . . It is with an emphasis on effective communication, through properly managed patient consultation sessions, that pharmacists can successfully engage in patient education and correct compliance related to problems that will lead to better treatment outcomes.
> (270)

The perspective recommended by Fisher (1992) needs to be tested by pharmacists engaged in patient education. However, his recommendation of an educational approach for his colleagues based on research and theory is an excellent starting point.

Similarly Fredette (1990) sought to base patient education on a theoretically defensible basis after becoming concerned that even after being taught, patients with cancer were often not well informed. Through striving to understand the problem more fully she proposed that the need for patients to adjust to having a serious illness must be built into any patient education programme. Fredette proposes educators must understand and facilitate the process of emotional adaptation within their teaching programmes:

> Understanding the nature of this process forms the basis for effective patient education since theories of adaptation describe behaviours that impact on motivation to learn, information required, and teaching methodology. Failure to attend to this variable of emotional response to the disease can prevent learning.
>
> (Fredette, 1990: 207)

The author proposes a six-step educational model drawing from the theories of Weisman (1979), Crate (1965), Engle (1964) and Kubler-Ross (1969) which is a valuable start to appreciating how adjustment to chronic illness could be allowed for when planning a teaching programme. Unfortunately the author has not presented any data to support the impact of the model in practice. Thus before this approach can be advocated research trials using it must be conducted. However, it is to her credit that she seeks to use a theoretically-based programme for patient education.

The need for nurse educators to develop the theoretical basis for their work has been called for before (Redman, 1993) and the issue will be discussed further in Chapter 8.

Conclusion

None of the models relating to patient education have yet been sufficiently used and tested to enable a body of research evidence to be developed to support them. Further work is needed before we will be able fully to understand and explain factors which influence health behaviour. However, what is important in the context of this book is to accept that patients choose whether to put information into practice and also that education to change behaviour must be multi-faceted; it is more than correcting a knowledge deficit. As no single factor can be said to ensure compliance it is unlikely that a single educational intervention could influence long-term behavioural change. There are different ways of viewing behavioural change, no single model is as yet supported by sufficient research to enable it to be accepted but it is important that work on this complex issue is being conducted.

KEY POINTS FROM CHAPTER 6

1 *Education to help people manage chronic health problems and illnesses is not a simple process*; many different factors are involved. As yet we do not understand which are the most important factors when trying to help individuals undertake self-management successfully. Failure to undertake prescribed or recommended actions to maintain health is commonplace and represents a major problem for both patients and the health care team.

2 *The terms compliance and non-compliance* are often used with regard to patients undertaking (or not undertaking) treatment regimens. At a time when we wish to encourage patients to be active participants in their health care, compliance is not considered an appropriate term.

3 *The relationship between knowledge and behaviour is not clear.* It is known that knowledge on its own will not lead to behavioural change, other factors must also be brought into play. The specific nature of these other factors is still a controversial issue.

4 *The complexity of the self-care regimen will have a bearing upon whether the patient feels able to follow it or not.* Patient educators must think carefully about what is being expected of patients. Patients must be consulted when regimens are drawn up and if a regimen appears too arduous steps to make it easier to follow should be taken. This would appear to be a very reasonable point and would foster partnership between patients and professionals, which was the philosophy proposed by Szasz and Hollender (1956) discussed in Chapter 1.

5   *Educators must accept that the perspectives of health profes-
    sionals and patients and clients can be quite different* (Cameron
    and Gregor, 1987). Self-management regimens will not be auto-
    matically accepted. Indeed they are often judged according to
    social rather than medical criteria (Strauss and Glaser, 1975).

6   *The work of Strauss and Glaser (1975) was presented* to help
    clarify why patients may not follow prescribed therapeutic regi-
    mens and illustrates that the regimen may be more troublesome
    than the illness itself.

7   *Different models aiming to explain or predict health manage-
    ment behaviour are presented,* for example the biomedical
    model, communication-based models, the Health Belief Model
    or the Stages of Change Model. These models serve to illus-
    trate that it is recognised across several disciplines that a variety
    of variables must be taken into account when seeking to modify
    health behaviour. Unfortunately, it is not clearly understood
    which models are most suitable in which situations. What the
    models do serve to illustrate however, is that patient education
    is not a simple, linear process. The models which are presented
    are still being applied, tested and debated.

8   *The quality of the interaction between the educator and the
    client is of vital importance* to the future success of a self-
    management regimen. The work of Cameron (1996) supports
    this perspective recommending a sensitive empathetic approach
    by the practitioner towards the patient. The work of Bartlett *et
    al.* (1984), Leventhal and Cameron (1987) and Ley (1988) all
    support the need for high-quality interaction/communication in
    patient education.

Chapter 7

Educational interventions to promote behavioural change

Introduction

In this chapter, the ways in which some of the issues and ideas discussed in Chapter 6 may be applied with the aim of helping people live with and successfully manage chronic health problems will be further examined. This chapter will concern educational interventions which have been designed to influence attitudes and beliefs in order to bring about and sustain behavioural change. As has been mentioned earlier in this book, it is important that educational practice should unite theory and research where possible. Different client groups may require quite different theoretical approaches, and one theoretical framework is unlikely to be suitable for all long-term self-management programmes. When searching the literature for appropriate research it is easy to become overwhelmed with a large variety of studies, involving different client groups, investigating different theoretical principles and variables and after reading widely to feel that no overall picture is emerging. For this reason, studies concerning educational programmes for people with rheumatoid disease, cancer and diabetes are the focus of this chapter. The studies in this chapter concern people with chronic health problems, as the needs of patients with more acute problems were considered in Chapters 4 and 5.

The terms psycho-education and multi-modal education have been coined to describe programmes in which a combination of interventions promote learning and psychological change. In Chapter 5 it was acknowledged that a single intervention is rarely successful; this would appear to be even more true for people with a chronic health condition. The use of psycho-education or multi-modal education amongst people diagnosed with rheumatoid disease or cancer will be considered and then the concept of empowerment will be discussed and, by way of an example, applied to people with diabetes. Finally, the research implications of the findings to date will be mentioned.

Psycho-education/multi-modal education

It would appear that a variety of interventions are required for patients with long-term health problems. The concern is that we do not know which of these interventions will be most appropriate to which individuals. In addition, according to Sluijs and Knibbe (1991), self-management behaviours are vastly different, and therefore a single theory is unlikely to explain and facilitate them all. Thus, health care providers must have a repertoire of skills which are theoretically-based if their educational interventions are to be effective.

Consider, for example, the implications of a regimen for a man who has just been diagnosed with hypertension. It is likely that he will be prescribed medication – possibly several tablets to be taken at different times – asked to lose weight and maintain a reduced weight, decrease salt intake, eat a low-fat diet, stop smoking, take more exercise and visit his health centre regularly to have his blood pressure monitored. The behaviours required to do all these things are quite different and may need different educational interventions to help the patient to achieve them all. Some will require knowledge acquisition, others, assertiveness, decision-making ability or communication skills if such an individual is to self-manage his hypertension effectively. An educational programme which only attends to one aspect of his learning needs would be too narrow to enable the totality of self-management to occur at an optimal level.

Sluijs and Knibbe (1991) found that educational strategies may need to be selected according to the length of time a patient is to sustain the behaviour. They suggested that education interventions based on behavioural therapy are helpful in the short term. However, for long-term change a self-regulation approach is advocated in which patients are active agents who choose their own goals and the behaviour to achieve them and evaluate progress. This approach stops patients from being passive or dependent on health professionals because it requires active participation of the patient or client. As a result of their analysis of research regarding different theoretical approaches to undertaking exercise as part of a medical regimen they were led to conclude that: 'Unplanned interventions are most likely to fail' (Sluijs and Knibbe, 1991: 201). This is an important point for all involved in patient education. So how should an educational programme be planned? Knowledge of appropriate literature seems to be an appropriate place to start.

Increasingly terms such as psycho-education and multi-modal interventions are used in the literature about the need for a repertoire of interventions rather than a single focus for education. Bernier (1992) describes psycho-education as: 'a broad range of cognitive, behavioural, and psychosocial interventions or treatment approaches that are combined for use with patients and families seeking or requiring information and social support at all stages of development in health and illness' (126).

Research work involving initiatives which could be termed 'psycho-education' will be considered below and are initially grouped according to the disease category with which the client group were diagnosed. By using the term psycho-education it is implicitly acknowledged that education is more than a 'bucket filling' exercise, that a patient-centred approach is preferable and furthermore, these interventions need to have some theoretical justification. The need for a structured psychological component to educational interventions is now widely supported (Basler, 1995). According to Jenkins (1995) the accumulating body of evidence in psychology suggests that:

> The cognitive aspects of education play an essential, but only a subsidiary, role in changing and maintaining behavioural habits. Studies of behaviour therapy and social learning theory have shown that values, motivational hierarchies, positive reinforcement, expectancies and social influences are critically important.
>
> (55)

Studies concerning people with rheumatoid disease

A considerable amount of high quality research has been undertaken to help understand the educational requirements and most appropriate interventions for people with a rheumatoid condition. Researchers in this clinical area are notable for the rigour of their developments: for example, the educational standards included in Chapter 5, and depth of inquiry in their investigations. This calibre of work helps to elevate patient education to treatment status, which, as has been discussed earlier, should be a goal for all patient educators.

Hawley (1995) considered psycho-educational interventions in the treatment of arthritis. She acknowledges that conventionally arthritis has been treated mainly through medication. However, in order to understand the medication and its side effects there has arisen a need for education. Hawley conducted an extensive review of 34 clinical trials dating from 1985–1995, relating to rheumatic disease. She clarified her understanding of the term psycho-education as:

> Psycho-educational intervention is the umbrella term that encompasses both traditional educational or teaching activities *and* psychological interventions. Many psycho-educational interventions combine an educational intervention and psychological intervention (e.g. behavioural therapy).
>
> (805)

Family and social support may also be involved. Thus the purpose is to influence outcomes by individuals voluntarily modifying behaviour and also to increase knowledge.

Hawley reports that she found that the interventions were difficult to evaluate due to differences in, for example, interventions, methods of sampling or follow-up times. For this reason meta-analysis of results was not possible. However, despite this problem, she concluded that psycho-educational interventions had a positive impact upon the management of arthritis and quality of life for clients. From the literature reviewed she detected improvements in 'pain, depressive symptoms, self-efficacy, coping abilities, and self-management behaviours such as exercise' (821).

Taal et al. (1996) conducted an interesting review to investigate whether a 'self-efficacy' approach to patient education could help promote self-management for people with rheumatic conditions. The aim of self-management is to relieve pain, prevent joint destruction, and preserve or improve function. Thus individuals with a rheumatic condition must have the knowledge and skills to strive to achieve these goals, plus they need problem-solving, decision-making and communication skills. Taal and colleagues selected Bandura's (1986) social learning theory as an appropriate theoretical framework to guide interventions and provide a detailed discussion of the way in which the theory is appropriate to these conditions.

Through a combination of standards set for arthritis patient education and the self-efficacy theory they propose criteria which should be included in self-management programmes and also feature in their evaluation. They are illustrated in Figure 7.1. They also state that this degree of initial planning is worthwhile because: 'The effectiveness of arthritis patient education depends heavily on the quality of planning' (236).

The analysis by Taal *et al.* provides an excellent example of the level of integration of theory with practice which is required if it is intended that educational interventions are grounded in theory. This work is included as a very good example of the way in which programmes need to be developed. However, Taal and colleagues did not report the value of the self-management programme. This is the crucial next step. While we must strive to develop a theoretical basis for educational interventions, their worth will only become known to us through use in practice. It is vital that we gain empirical evidence to support whether or not these interventions work, in terms of helping patients achieve their stated learning outcomes.

An interesting review was conducted by DeVellis and Blalock (1993) who critically analysed the value of psychological and educational interventions to reduce disability for people with arthritis. They acknowledged that most psycho-educational programmes comprise

---

1 A thorough problem analysis.

2 The use of a theoretical model.

3 An attempt to influence knowledge, behaviour and health status.

4 An attempt to teach effective self-management skills.

5 The use of effective methods of teaching self-management skills and strengthening self-efficacy appraisals.

6 The involvement of people from the patient's social environment (spouse, close relatives).

7 A proper evaluation of the programme's effectiveness.

Figure 7.1   Key points to be included in a self-management programme guided by social learning theory

several parts and that it is important to evaluate the components of a programme rather than a total programme. They suggested that the giving of general information to clients should only be a small part of a 'multi-intervention strategy'. After considering many studies they reported that providing educational information on its own will not have a beneficial impact on the self-management of arthritis. They evaluated the following four categories of intervention:

Illness self-management skills – such as the use of heat and massage to manage pain. The data examined by DeVellis and Blalock suggested that: 'in the context of an educational or psychological intervention, training patients to use these techniques to manage their arthritis is of unknown benefit' (402).

Biofeedback – such as to develop skills to relax muscles in response to a signal that corresponds to a biological process – was evaluated. They report that overall such strategies have some benefit but only as part of a programme of care. The results do not warrant use of biofeedback alone.

Cognitive-behavioural techniques – this involves the use of procedures to divert attention away from pain and to increase skills to solve everyday problems. Overall, there is evidence to support the use of cognitive-behavioural therapies to develop positive changes in people with arthritis in the short term. Longer-term, or sustained change was not evident, leading to the conclusion that single interventions are not enough but that sustained therapy may be needed.

Social support – such interventions encouraged patients to develop supportive relationships to help them manage their arthritis. However, in terms of a research basis for practice there was 'little evidence that providing opportunities for social support yields consistent benefits for arthritis patients' (408). However, the authors stress that this must be distinguished from naturally occurring help from family and friends. Support is interpreted as more than contact but what is beneficial is not yet fully understood.

The authors conclude their report by suggesting that we need to give greater attention to individual assessment to understand how arthritis influences each person and their lifestyle and vice versa.

Thus no single educational intervention was considered to improve quality of life for people with arthritis indicating that a multi-dimensional approach is required. This form of analysis is very useful to the profession, because it is only when we have access to this sort of information that we can start to sift through interventions and find those which can be justified and those which cannot.

The findings from this review also provide food for thought for nurses working in other situations in which chronic illness is the major cause of ill health. Analysis of research results such as that provided by DeVellis and Blalock (1993) reminds us that the outcomes of different types of interventions must be evaluated and their worth in practice quantified when possible. It is likely that patients with other chronic health problems will also need to experience a variety of educational interventions rather than any single form of intervention.

Studies concerning people with cancer

A considerable body of work relating to the educational needs of people with cancer has developed over the past 20 years. Drawing from this Devine and Westlake (1995) conducted a meta-analysis of 116 studies published between 1976 and 1993. The purpose of the study was to investigate the effects of 'psychoeducational care on psychological well-being, and cancer related knowledge about one's health condition in adults with cancer' (1370).

For the purposes of their analysis psycho-educational interventions are reported to include; 'instruction about cancer, cancer treatment and living with cancer; counseling and therapy and behavioural approaches' (1369). As a result of their investigation it was concluded that statistically significant beneficial effects of psycho-educational interventions were found for the seven outcomes of: anxiety, depression, mood, nausea, vomiting, pain and knowledge. Thus this work lends support to the need for multiple educational interventions, but they follow this by stating that further research is required to explore whether some types of intervention are better than others. They recommend that nurses should evaluate whether their own practice includes psycho-educational care and the extent to which it is based on research findings.

The work of Fawzy (1995) with people newly diagnosed with cancer also supports the need for psycho-educational interventions, recognising that a diagnosis of cancer usually causes psychological distress. A structured programme including health education, stress management, behavioural training, coping and psycho-social group support was developed and tested. She reports how the programme was developed from research-based evidence which indicated that several modes, when used singly, had something to offer people with cancer: 'It seemed logical therefore, that if the effective elements were combined, the resulting comprehensive intervention would prove even more powerful in affecting the desired outcomes' (235).

The intervention, which she reports in detail, was used with people recently diagnosed with malignant melanoma which was treated surgically. The people were then randomised to a control group receiving routine medical care (34 people) or to an experimental group receiving standard care, plus the intervention (34 people). Fawzy reports that after a six-year follow-up, in addition to significantly more positive feedback relating to affective state, immune function and quality of life amongst the experimental group, these differences in mortality and morbidity were apparent:

> For the control group, there was a trend towards recurrence (13/34) and a statistically significant greater rate of death (10/34) than for the experimental patients (7/34 and 3/34), respectively.
>
> (237)

These results appear to justify the initial outlay in terms of time and resources to run the programme.

Mirolo et al. (1994) tested a combined educational intervention to help patients self-manage lymphoedema after surgery and/or radiotherapy to treat breast cancer. The study involved 25 people who had lymphoedema for at least five years. The intervention involved intensive treatment involving massage, compression bandaging and sequential pneumatic compression plus an educational programme to 'provide skills in exercise, massage, bandage and containment garment use' (197). As a result of their study they report that their multiple intervention of physical therapy plus self-management education reduced the lymphoedema, decreased the need for physical help, and maintained quality of life immediately post-intervention and for up to 12 months at the last follow-up. This is an example of a mixed intervention which both increased knowledge in relation to self-management of the problem and also in terms of self-esteem and body image which were components of the quality of life measures.

The reports of Fawzy (1995) and Mirolo and colleagues (1995) lend weight to the view that education should not be separated from the clinical management of a condition, a point which is recommended by Jenkins (1995). Furthermore, after acknowledging the importance of multiple educational interventions, we still need to know which interventions are most useful and in which situations. This information would enable nurses to prioritise the range of interventions offered, which is particularly important when pressed for time in which to teach. It is likely that the general principles underpinning the results mentioned above can be applied to those with other health care problems, although ideally, their effects should be evaluated in practice.

Facilitating empowerment – a psycho-educational intervention

In this section the concept of empowerment will be considered because its promotion requires psychological and educational interventions and also because it is currently in vogue. This possibly has more to do with its being politically attractive (because, notionally, self-reliance and self-care are a potential means of easing the burden of care from the state to individuals (Chavasse, 1992)), than with its potential beneficial effects upon patients.

Promoting empowerment may be considered as a form of psycho-education because its goals are to help people to live with health problems (although as a concept it is not confined to health care). Rodwell (1996), who conducted a thorough analysis of the concept, defines empowerment as 'a process of transferring power' which 'includes the development of a positive self-esteem and recognition of the worth of self and others' (307).

Empowerment occurs as part of an educational process in which individuals appreciate their power in a situation and their ability to make decisions: 'The individual has the power and freedom to make choices and to accept responsibility for actions. . . . Empowerment involves a partnership and mutual decision-making' (Rodwell, 1996: 309).

Furthermore, it is generally accepted that: 'Health professionals cannot empower people, people can only empower themselves' (310).

In such an educational programme intangible concepts such as autonomy, responsibility, accountability and authority are the focus. It is difficult to work with abstract variables, difficult to teach them and, perhaps crucially for the empowerment approach, extremely difficult to evaluate them. However, health professionals can and do design programmes in which individuals can be facilitated to empower themselves. This form of psycho-education will be illustrated with reference to the education of people with diabetes.

In an acknowledgement that knowledge alone will not necessarily result in improved control of diabetes, Anderson *et al.* (1995) conducted a study to investigate if a programme to increase patient empowerment could lead to improved control. Patients, who were initially self-selected in that they responded to an advert seeking volunteers, were randomly assigned to an intervention group and a 'wait-listed' control group. The control group were used as a comparison against which to measure the intervention group but were then offered the empowerment programme and they were also then used to compare pre- and post-intervention changes. The study was designed to achieve the following objectives:

1   enhance the ability of patients to identify and set realistic goals;
2   apply a systematic problem-solving process to eliminate barriers to achieving these goals;
3   cope with circumstances that cannot be changed;
4   manage the stress caused by living with diabetes as well as the general stress of daily life;
5   identify and obtain appropriate social support;
6   improve their ability to be self-motivated.

(Anderson *et al.*, 1995: 944)

Undoubtedly, all those involved needed sufficient knowledge and skills to be able to manage their diabetes on a daily basis. This study was designed to help the information to be better utilised. The programme consisted of six two-hourly sessions, one per week for six weeks. Pre- and post-measures of self-efficacy relating to the above listed objectives were taken and diabetes control was evaluated via blood results from pre-, post- and follow-up blood samples. The follow-up measures were taken six weeks after completion of the programme. The results, based on a sample of 64 patients indicated that the 'intervention group showed gains over the control group on four of the eight self-efficacy subscales and two of the five diabetes attitude subscales' (943). The blood glucose results also improved significantly after the empowerment programme. The authors conclude that:

> patient empowerment is an effective approach to developing educational interventions for addressing psychosocial aspects of living with diabetes. Furthermore, patient empowerment is conducive to improving blood glucose control. In an ideal setting, patient education would address equally blood glucose management and the psychosocial challenges of living with diabetes.
>
> (943)

These results are encouraging, but it should be remembered that six weeks is not a very long follow-up time when dealing with a life-long condition. This study would have greater weight if blood glucose levels were still improved in the experimental group a year later.

This study would support the philosophy of Szasz and Hollender (1956) discussed in Chapter 1, that in chronic health care situations patients and professionals need to work together as partners with shared power and responsibility. Programmes to increase patients' power and confidence will help this philosophy to be achieved. Funnell et al. (1990) offer an interesting comparison between a traditional medically orientated approach to patient education and an empowering approach in which the need for partnership is clearly illustrated. It is shown in Figure 7.2.

According to Feste and Anderson (1995) empowerment involves helping patients to be aware of their own health values, needs and goals. The traditional compliance-based model of instruction must be relinquished. The education is not just to ensure that patients follow treatment but that they are in the position to make the choices about their health that best suit their needs.

Feste and Anderson (1995) state that: 'Being empowered means that patients have learned enough about disease and health to judge the cost benefits of adopting a wide variety of healthcare recommendations' (140). To facilitate empowerment health professionals must adopt a reversal of their usual way of providing education and put the patient in the driving seat. The interventions are used to help the individual decide how they wish to manage their health rather than imposing a schedule upon them. Feste and Anderson

Traditional medical model	Empowering person-centred model
Diabetes is a physical illness	Diabetes is a bio-psycho-social illness
Relationship of educator to patient is authoritarian based on professional expertise	Relationship of educator and patient is democratic and based on shared expertise
Problems and learning needs are usually defined by the professional	Problems and learning needs are usually identified by the patient
Professional is viewed as problem solver and caregiver, responsible for diagnosis, treatment and outcome	Patient is viewed as problem solver and caregiver, professional acts as a resource, both share responsibility for treatment decisions and outcome
Goal is compliance with recommendations. Behavioural strategies are used to increase compliance with recommended treatment. A lack of compliance is viewed as a failure of patient and provider	Goal is to enable patients to make informed choices. Behavioural strategies are used to help patients change behaviours of their choosing. A lack of goal achievement is viewed as feedback and used to modify goals and strategies
Behaviour changes are externally motivated	Behaviour changes are internally motivated
Patient is powerless relative to professional	Patient and professional have power

Figure 7.2   Key differences between traditional and empowering educational models
Source: Slightly modified from Funnell *et al.*, 1990: 39

suggest the points in Figure 7.3 as ways to help facilitate the development of empowerment.

This form of education is quite different to one which dwells upon knowledge. Clearly people need knowledge, but an empowerment philosophy is to help people modify behaviour and feel in control of their health needs.

Empowerment has also been usefully applied in relation to other client groups, for example with the elderly through carefully refined

1   *wellbeing* is defined in a way that encourages people to identify their own values, needs and goals;

2   *people are encouraged to assess their own self-image* and consider practical ways by which it could be improved if desired;

3   *motivation* is examined to help raise individuals' awareness of the internal and external influences upon their decisions;

4   *adaptability* is encouraged as it is this which helps people to adjust to the changes which need to be made in the course of living with a chronic condition;

5   *stress*: people are encouraged to examine the sources of stress in their lives and how they cope with it. Identification of means to deal with stress may increase ability to cope;

6   *problem-solving* is promoted and taught as a step by step process. This skill can help people overcome the problems they face when living with a chronic illness;

7   *means of support are identified*; types of support which suit them best and how they can get it are discussed.

Figure 7.3 Strategies to facilitate the development of empowerment

communication strategies (Le May, 1998). Anderson (1995) points out that the traditional model of medical care is best suited to acutely ill, highly dependent patients, as has been discussed previously when looking at the philosophy proposed by Szasz and Hollender (1956). He goes on to argue that this approach is then internalised to the extent that it is assumed that it is the appropriate approach for all kinds of patient care:

> A major result of the traditional medical approach to care is that medical students, residents, and other physician trainees are taught that they will be in charge of and responsible for the treatment of illness.
>
> (413)

However, he argues that in chronic illness situations this approach is unsuitable, and indeed is likely to be at the root of the compliance/

non-compliance problem. If we do not presume that patients should do as they are told, but rather that they are provided with information and skills to enable them to manage themselves, then they cannot be labelled 'disobedient' (non-compliant) if they then decide to manage their condition in their own way, because it was never suggested that they should 'obey' in the first place. This represents a shift in the way we view patient education. As Anderson (1995: 413) comments:

> Patient education has been viewed by many as an attempt to extend and increase the influence of health care professionals on the behaviour of their patients. Patient empowerment, on the other hand, attempts to enhance patients' ability to influence their own lives by helping them learn how to make informed choices about the care of their diabetes.

Although he is addressing people with diabetes in this case, the same argument could be applied to many other chronic conditions, as it is widely recognised that non-compliance is a problem which influences the management of a very wide range of health problems. Building on his work these recommendations are made: that health care professionals accept that the daily management of health problems is carried out by the patients, and therefore the focus of care and education should be to enable patients to make informed decisions about their self-management; that pejorative terms such as compliance are no longer used; that training schools include paradigms for care which are suitable for individuals with chronic illness conditions; making health professionals mentors, coaches and advisors rather than controllers; and finally, to help patients have a clearer understanding of their own role in their treatment and their relationships with health care professionals. So, although the case for patient empowerment was made with reference to those with diabetes, it is considered that many other people with a chronic health problem could benefit from such an approach, although as always, this assumption needs to be tested in practice.

The need for co-ordinated research relating to the self-management of chronic illness

Cameron and Best (1987) reviewed literature relating to adherence to health behaviour change programmes and found that the existing literature lacked coherence and direction. Overall there was little sense of a 'systematic accumulation of knowledge' (149). They recommend that we need to be more organised theoretically and to strive to plan interventions based on empirically-based behavioural principles. The studies presented above would support the need for programmes of research to be conducted in which theories and ideas are tested so that a cohesive picture of the situation and a body of knowledge can emerge. This sentiment would be supported by Leventhal and Cameron (1987).

Bernier (1992), while suggesting that psycho-education should be more widely applied in educational contexts, also emphasises the need for greater use of experimental and quasi-experimental research designs to develop theory and practice in patient education. As Assal *et al.* (1983: 1) have reported: 'Since we are deeply convinced that teaching patients is an essential part of treatment, we have to examine the teaching process as systematically as biochemical pathways or the pharmacology of a drug.'

How often in nursing do we apply this degree of rigour to patient teaching? It is only through the results of experimental research that educators will be able to defend their work in teaching patients and justify the time, money and resources which are required to conduct effective teaching. Fain (1995) acknowledges the difficulties that practitioners face when attempting to undertake research to provide a research base and validate practice, yet reports that regardless of difficulties research must be the basis for practice. When looking at nursing in the new health care environment Sines (1995) warns that nurses will need to be able to articulate and market their contribution to health care and to co-ordinate and plan their care with others. If adequate resources are to be channelled into patient education nurses must be able to demonstrate that their work is research-based and effective.

While accepting that greater consistency of approach to research is required it is also important to ensure that, when appropriate research is available, the results are used. As Sluijs and Knibbe (1991: 191) report, unfortunately: 'Health care providers seldom act according to the recommendations derived from research findings.'

In Chapter 2 the need for evidence-based practice in the current health care climate was emphasised, thus nurses must strive to base their teaching on research-based principles where possible.

Conclusion

Literature consistently supports the unfortunate situation that the majority of patients/clients do not undertake self-management of long-term health problems even if the consequences of not doing so are potentially life threatening. Whilst patients are not obliged to 'do as they are told', if the goal of patient education is behaviour change (as many believe), then many patient education interventions are unsuccessful and thus cannot be considered effective nor efficient. From the wide range of material, representing a diversity of clinical needs, client groups and research methods, the need for educational programmes to include a psychological component consistently emerges.

In this chapter, the ideas put forward in Chapter 6 to help meet the educational needs of people with chronic illnesses have been followed through with application to three client groups. As the volume of detailed research-based literature burgeons there appears to be merit in seeking research-based work relevant to particular client groups when seeking to identify appropriate theoretical frameworks to inform educational practice. The work of people such as DeVellis and Blalock (1993), Hawley (1995) and Devine and Westlake (1995) demonstrate the value of reviewing literature relating to a particular client group in determining what tactics are likely to be useful in constructing an educational approach. Thus nurses working in cancer care, for example, should focus their literature reviews on this clinical area rather than consulting a wide spectrum of work which is likely to be overwhelmingly broad.

The emphasis of an educational intervention will need to vary according to individual assessment results. There may be no such thing as a totally standardised package of information for patients with diagnosed diseases, but it is probable that patients belonging to a particular client group will have some areas of common need. Appreciation of appropriate research may enable practitioners to learn of interventions to help improve the degree to which individuals are able to self-manage their health problems, rather than simply knowing about them. While there is merit in investigating the needs of clients as a group, at a practice level we must still think about the needs of each person first and the medical condition second.

KEY POINTS FROM CHAPTER 7

1   *The importance of careful assessment of patients' educational needs has been a recurring theme.* This includes more than identification of a knowledge deficit, it also includes views and perceptions about self-managing their health or treatment regimen, support systems and lifestyle. An individualised, holistic approach appears to be a more effective strategy than 'providing vast amounts of standardised information, (Frederikson, 1995: 237). The provision of information alone will often not help the goals of education to be achieved when patients have a long-term health problem. Building on this knowledge possible ways in which self-management of medical regimens and health problems can be facilitated have been considered.

2   *A single theory to explain the relationship between knowledge and health behaviour* is unlikely adequately to serve a diversity of patient education situations. Thus health care providers must have a repertoire of skills which are theoretically based if their educational interventions are to be effective (Sluijs and Knibbe, 1991). Use of theory and research is vital in patient education and must be informed by literature relating to the relevant client group.

3   *Research indicates that single interventions will not facilitate long-term change* and that ongoing education and support is required (Bernier, 1992). A programme of educational intervention appropriate to the needs of the client group and modified for individual use may lead to more realistic interventions in the long term.

4   *Time and effort spent on educational preparation may reap rewards* in terms of the promotion of self-management of health programmes in the longer term.

5   *The use of psycho-educational or multi-modal interventions in patient education* has been discussed and supported, with particular reference to people with rheumatoid disease or with cancer.

6   *Empowering patients may enable them to become more active in the management of their own problems* which may eventually lead to improved health outcomes. Examples of how the process of empowerment may be conducted were included with reference to people with diabetes.

7   *Despite the information which is available, patient educators do not usually use the results of research as a basis for their interventions* (Sluijs and Knibbe, 1991). Patient educators must be as well prepared for patient education as for any other field of practice. *Ad hoc* patient teaching is unlikely to be successful: 'Unplanned interventions are most likely to fail' (Sluijs and Knibbe, 1991: 201). Therefore nurses involved in patient education must be adequately prepared to undertake this activity in order to maximise opportunities to be effective.

Chapter 8

Nurses as educators of patients and clients

Introduction

Since this book has been directed chiefly at nurses, it may be thought to be implicit within the book that nurses are the ideal people to undertake patient education. In Chapters 1 and 6 it was noted that care for those with a chronic illness represents the vast majority of the health care required today. All people with a chronic condition will require a minimum of some information, while others will benefit from extensive education programmes which may well involve cognitive, psychomotor and attitudinal dimensions in order to undertake self-management effectively.

Someone has to equip such people with the necessary skills and know-how to be confidently self-caring. Equally important are the needs of people with acute health problems who are likely to need education and support to help them to cope. *Someone* has to provide appropriate education to meet patients' short-term and acute needs. However, it may be that other professional and non-professional groups have claims which are equal to those of nurses to be the sole or chief providers of patient education. Although a detailed examination of these possibly competing claims is outside the scope of this book, they will be briefly discussed below.

In the bulk of this chapter, however, the specific case for the use of nurses as patient educators will be examined. Points which appear to support the case that nurses should be patient educators and also factors which may mitigate them adequately fulfilling this role will be discussed. The feasibility of their role in patient education in the current health care climate will be discussed and the implications of them not undertaking this role will be considered. Finally, the need for evidence-based practice will be revisited, building on points made in Chapter 2.

Provision of patient education – why nurses?

Lay educators?

Having noted that someone should provide patient education, it may be felt that this someone should be a health professional, since they ought to have a more appropriate knowledge base, professional network and communication skills than the general public. If they do not we must very critically challenge their pre-registration programmes. Some lay people may have developed extensive expertise related to a particular condition; for example, individuals with a stoma may themselves become experts in stoma care and be a valuable source of education to fellow patients.

However, there is no professional safeguard associated with such people. There is no means of regulating the standards and accuracy of the information delivered. It is a bit like the argument, 'Would you go to a State Registered Chiropodist rather than a Chiropodist?'. It is only by attending a State Registered Chiropodist that the public can be assured that the person claiming expertise has successfully completed an approved preparatory programme. Unqualified teachers have no professional accountability for their actions as all is done in good faith. How could the public be protected from charlatans? Where would be the protection from myths and 'old wives tales'? To what extent would the information be anecdotal rather than research-based? This is not to imply that lay educators do operate in this way; it is only to illustrate that there is no protection for patients if they should choose to do so. Similarly, professional registration does not necessarily protect the public from rogue professionals, but does, at least, provide a transparent account of what standards members of the profession are expected to meet. One crucial element of such standards, in nursing, is the increasing duty to base care on the best available evidence.

Undeniably, there is an important role for lay teachers and also for patient support groups (Visser and Herbert, 1994). However, while lay teachers can provide valuable peer support they should only be an adjunct to teaching rather than the sole providers.

Professional health educators/promoters

Very detailed debate about the concepts of patient education, health education and health promotion regularly takes place to clarify the remit and function of these activities and the people who undertake them. As yet there does not appear to be a consensus of opinion about a definition of these activities or by whom they should be undertaken (Caraher, 1998; van Eijk, 1998).

In the move to shift health promotion from a medically dominated model of intervention, it could be argued that doctors, nurses or physiotherapists for example, may not be the most suitable breeds of professionals to undertake this role. Rather, that health promotion could be undertaken by individuals specifically prepared for their role, who will look beyond disease and give greater emphasis to social and political factors which influence health needs. Throughout this book the explicit focus has been patient education for people with a diagnosed health problem, rather than health promotion at a primary prevention level such as healthy lifestyle advice. When focusing on patients with an acknowledged health problem the need for patient education from professionals in the health care situation, with appropriate knowledge of disease processes and treatment, as well as an understanding of health, should be beyond dispute.

Other health professionals in patient education

Doctors can, and of course do, provide patient education. However, the literature demonstrates quite clearly that whilst they have a sufficient knowledge base to enable them to educate patients they rarely have the time and may not have the necessary communication skills, nor for some the inclination, to educate patients effectively (Breemhaar et al., 1996; Arborelius and Osterberg, 1995; Calnan, 1995; Skelton et al., 1995; Audit Commission, 1993; Wallace, 1986). Of course, the same could be said of nurses.

Dieticians, physiotherapists, occupational therapists, pharmacists, indeed all health professionals, have a remit to undertake patient education. All these professionals should be involved in patient education, but they often have a very specific role rather than adopting a holistic approach to care. For example, dieticians are likely to confine their educational input to matters relating to diet, chiropodists to the feet. If patient education were to be delivered by one specialist or professional group after another there is a danger that it could be fragmented and uncoordinated. In addition to specialist input there needs to be a general and all-inclusive basis for patient education.

Theoretical and professional justification for nurses as patient educators

Only doctors and nurses have a remit to consider entire individuals, and of these professions, nurses claim to have the wider brief because rather than focusing mainly on physiological aspects of illness nurses claim also to attend to spiritual, psychological and social issues. Theoretically then, nurses are well placed to be key players in the process of patient education, drawing in other health professionals as required. Perhaps the strongest, but not necessarily the most easily justified argument is that they are the largest group of health care workers, so by virtue of their numbers they should be able to do more patient education than any other group (Smith, 1979; Pender, 1996). Undeniably nurses make up the greatest portion of the workforce (Tierney, 1993). As McKenna (1995), drawing from several sources, reports:

> In the United Kingdom (UK) nurses currently make up approximately 70% of the health service work force, and they cost 40% of total health service expenditure, 60% of the total health service pay bill and they command 3% of the public purse.
>
> (452)

Being the predominant portion of the workforce alone would not justify their position as key players in patient education; however, there are also other reasons to support nurses as patient educators to add strength to the argument. In a hospital setting nurses have extended contact with patients as they provide 24-hour continuous care (Syred, 1981). They have very close, possibly the closest, contact with patients, thus nurses have more opportunities to teach than other professionals. Drawing from literature published in the 1970s and 1980s, Close (1988) suggests that nurses are in an ideal position to assess patients' learning needs during the course of their initial and ongoing patient assessments and they are often the first people the patient approaches for information. Nurses have an appropriate bio-psycho-social knowledge base and expertise to inform their teaching (Pender, 1996). It can also be said that patient education is required if total care needs are to be met. Therefore, if nurses wish to continue to be regarded as providers of holistic care, this activity must be part of their remit.

Nurses are often at the centre of the care process so they are in an ideal position to co-ordinate education of patients by the whole health care team, peers and support groups as necessary. In addition nurses frequently help patients to interpret information given to them by other professionals (Busby and Gilchrist, 1992) and help them to formulate appropriate questions when referred to other professionals. There is some support for the view that health professionals (including nurses) and patients believe that patient education is a part of nursing care (Pohl, 1965; Honan et al., 1988; Coonrod et al., 1994), although Tilley et al. (1987) report that while patients recognise that nurses are a source of education they would prefer to be taught by their doctor. Lisper et al. (1997) also found that patients preferred to receive information about medication from their doctor. However, this may be due to nurses not being perceived as having the necessary competence to teach, as has been pointed out by Winslow (1976, cited by Jenny, 1978: 347):

> most patients do not see me in a teaching role until I demonstrate my competence and ability to fulfil their teaching needs; then they ask many questions and rely heavily on me for the information.

If nurses were confident when teaching, patients might then prefer them to be the key players in patient education.

Nurse theorists support the case that nurses have a role to play in patient education (Peplau, 1952; Henderson, 1966; Orem, 1985; Benner, 1984). Moreover, statutory bodies such as the General Nursing Council for England and Wales and the National Board for Nursing Midwifery and Health Visiting have traditionally endorsed the role of nurses in patient education (Close, 1988). The Code of Professional Conduct issued by the United Kingdom Central Council for Nurses, Midwives and Health Visitors advises that nurses must: 'ensure that no action or omission on [her] part . . . is detrimental to the interests, condition or safety of patients or clients' (UKCC, 1992: 5).

This can be interpreted as support for nurses' involvement in patient education, for if nurses neglect to teach patients (for example, about the need to fast prior to an operation or the need to take their medicine when they are discharged home) then the consequences could be detrimental to patients' health.

Research into the subject of patient education has also endorsed the role for nurses in this activity. For example, the study by Smith et al. (1997) which revealed that 40 per cent of older people felt they had not received enough information about their condition in hospital led the authors to conclude that: 'Nurses are in a strong position to ensure patients are kept well informed and fully understand what is being said to them and to ensure that the information needs of the most frail patients are met' (53).

Thus from organisational, professional, traditional and current perspectives it appears that the case for nurses to be key players in patient education can be justified. Only rarely has the involvement of nurses in patient education been directly challenged (Luker and Caress, 1989), although it has been indirectly challenged through reports in which nurses are not fulfilling their potential, as will be discussed later in this chapter.

Clarifying the role of nurses in patient education

Having found considerable evidence to support the involvement of nurses in patient education it is important to clarify the nature of this role and from the literature this role is by no means clearly understood. Redman (1993) suggested the following goals relating to patient education which institutions should aim to provide:

1   support the development of the client, and keep untoward side-effects of the education to a minimum;
2   balance client's definition of needs with those of the institution;
3   provide access to its special skills by those who need it.

These are very broad goals and relate to educational functions of institutions overall rather than specifically to nurses, so their input remains undefined. However, if institutions state intended goals in relation to patient education it is a start, as nurses can then determine, with other health care professionals, what is their specific contribution to these goals.

The work of Benner (1984) is more helpful in terms of attempting to clarify nurses' contribution to patient education. When examining nursing activity she identified a teaching-coaching function as one of seven domains of nursing practice as follows:

• The helping role
• **The teaching-coaching function**
• The diagnostic and patient monitoring function

- Effective management of rapidly changing situation
- Administering and monitoring therapeutic interventions and regimens
- Monitoring and ensuring the quality of health care practices
- Organisational and work-role competencies

(Benner, 1984: 46)

She suggests that:

> nurses become expert at coaching a patient through an illness. They take what is foreign and fearful to the patient and make it familiar and thus less frightening. Teaching and learning transactions require great skill under the best of circumstances, but they take on new demands and require different skills when the learner is threatened or ill.
>
> (77–78)

This is an important contribution to clarifying what could be a realistic yet valuable role for nurses in patient education. From her analysis of nursing activity, Benner defines competencies within the teaching-coaching function and they are illustrated in Figure 8.1.

Benner also acknowledges that these competencies probably represent only a fraction of all the teaching-coaching competencies

---

- Timing: capturing a patient's readiness to learn.

- Assisting patients to integrate the implications of illness and recovery into their lifestyles.

- Eliciting and understanding the patient's interpretation of his/her illness.

- Providing an interpretation of the patient's condition and giving a rationale for procedures.

- The coaching function: making culturally avoided aspects of an illness approachable and understandable.

Figure 8.1   Benner's teaching-coaching competencies
Source: Benner, 1984

unique to nursing in an acute setting. However, work such as this is important, even if it is incomplete, because it provides a basis from which nurses can analyse the scope of their patient education role. It should be noted that Benner presents a picture of nurses in acute rather than chronic situations and of how an expert rather than a novice nurse may be expected to undertake this role. The issue of level of expertise required to undertake patient education successfully will be returned to later in this chapter.

Wilson-Barnett and Osborne (1983) also attempted to clarify the nature of the nurse's role in patient education. They evaluated 29 reports on patient teaching and drew out implications for nursing practice. Drawing from the literature reviewed they suggested that types of teaching which nurses could include in their repertoire of skills would include:

1   attempt to provide patients with information related to their particular worries prior to stressful events such as surgery;
2   prepare patients for life at home when convalescing;
3   help patients understand their illness and disease.

The authors go on to state: 'These topics should not really need special knowledge. . . . Much of this teaching needs to be orientated to patients' feelings, concerns and experiences; technical topics are less relevant to their needs' (42).

All nurses should be capable of undertaking this level of intervention: they must know enough about illness and disease to be providing the care for the patients in the first place, they should be orientated to the place of work, know the names and responsibilities of colleagues and the nature of the investigations for which they prepare patients, and be able to relay this information to help reduce stress generated by being in an unfamiliar place facing an unknown procedure. Currently, hospital-based nurses need to help prepare patients for discharge and involve community personnel to provide care, including on-going education as necessary, if the currently fashionable concept of the 'seamless' service is to be achieved. Nurses must be good communicators both verbally and non-verbally as this skill is a vital part of all dimensions of their work. Indeed there is evidence to suggest that many nurses are already involved in this form of activity (Latter et al., 1992). However, the situation does get more complicated as patients' needs become progressively more acute or chronic.

In Chapters 6 and 7, the particular needs of people with chronic health problems were discussed. The educational needs of these people are quite different from those in an acute situation. To help clarify what forms of educational interventions may be required, Dunn (1995) suggests an educational continuum (not specifically relating to nurses) which may help meet the needs of different client groups (see Figure 8.2).

A similar continuum for nursing interventions in patient education could be developed to clarify the nature of nursing educational skills required for nurses to be effectively involved in this activity (see Figure 8.3).

This is not presented as a complete or static picture, but to illustrate that patient education is not a narrow activity, rather it spans a diversity of interventions. Different strategies will be required by different individuals who may have a similar medical condition but who have different personal circumstances and abilities. Nurses in differing situations, both clinical and geographical, need to clarify what they believe the scope of their practice should be and what they can realistically offer patients. All nurses do not need to be skilled at all interventions. As with other aspects of care, there will be some activities which require more expertise than others. This then needs to be confirmed at managerial levels and by other relevant members of the health care team to ensure that a valuable and

Acute illness consultation:	Traditional clinical interview
	Information-gathering skills
	Focus on pathophysiology
	Short-term intervention
Chronic illness consultation:	Patient–doctor communication
	Information-gathering skills
	Focus on behavioural skills
	Short-term with follow-up
Chronic illness management:	Human behaviour change
	Information-sharing skills
	Focus on relationship
	Long-term intervention

Figure 8.2 Continuum of illness interventions for medical professions

Acute health problems

Assessment according to physiological status

As appropriate:-

Information-giving – minimal if condition necessitates e.g. basics about surroundings, events, immediate treatment.

Enough for patient to give informed consent to treatment if condition sufficiently stable, if not, transfer information-giving to next of kin.

Increase amount of information according to wishes and capabilities of patient.

Prioritise teaching to avoid overloading patient.

Keep family informed.

Interventions to alleviate anxiety e.g. reassurance, continuity of care, presence of nurse, providing realistic accounts of what will occur.

Documentation of patient education.

Chronic health problems

Assessment of need to identify patients' learning needs and relevant factors influencing this process.

As appropriate:-

Verbal information/teaching.

Written information, selected material to supplement verbal teaching.

Demonstration/instruction of new skills.

Supplementary educational interventions e.g. audio-visual, computer-based.

Plan for ongoing support.

Development of rapport.

Changing roles to facilitate patient having a more active role.

Relinquishing control of health to patient.

Encouraging behavioural change by being aware of the importance of health care regimens fitting into existing lifestyle rather than vice versa.

Accept that patient has the right to choose nature of actions.

Co-ordination of teaching by other health professionals.

Involve patient support and peer groups as appropriate.

Acknowledgement of the influence of psychological/social/political factors influencing care.

Investment in the human relationship in the management of chronic illness.

Documentation of patient education.

Figure 8.3   Possible continuum for nursing interventions in patient education

comprehensive service is available to patients. Tilley and colleagues (1987) also stress the need for nurses to define their area of responsibility in patient education and make the following suggestion:

> Nurse practitioners and nurse educators should work to define that body of knowledge which is the nurse's unique responsibility to teach patients. Rather than providing medically-oriented information, the nurse's role may be to provide assistance to patients with interpreting their illness experience and integrating the implications of that experience into their lifestyle.
>
> (Tilley *et al.*, 1987: 299)

As nurses work in a wide range of situations it is unlikely that a single definition of responsibility will cover all nurses. However, it is important that they clarify their goals in relation to patient education as this is the starting point for all further activity. Only when the remit of patient education is more clearly understood will it be possible for nurses to own this area of practice, to set standards and to ensure that their work is research-based as far as is possible and that it is of demonstrable value to patients and their families. They can then identify what resources they need and what preparation and access to other specialists will be required. By undertaking an analysis of their role and forward planning to undertake it, research would suggest that teaching will be more efficient and effective. Time spent on unplanned, uncoordinated, ill-defined educational goals will, in the long run, be a poor use of nursing time and offer an inadequate and fragmented service to patients.

Are nurses fulfilling their role as patient educators?

Having considered the potential remit of nurses in patient education it is pertinent to investigate the extent to which nurses are fulfilling their role as patient educators. Latter *et al.* (1992) investigated the perceived practice of health education in acute settings across England. Although they used the term health education it was defined to include five types of activity: patient education, information-giving, healthy lifestyle advice, encouraging patient participation and encouraging family participation. The vast majority of wards across

Activity	Percentage of wards nationally reported to be involved – they 'always' or 'sometimes' include the activity in practice	
	%	n
Patient education	86	(2253)
Information-giving	83	(2184)
Healthy lifestyle advice	78	(2063)
Encouraging patient participation	71	(1854)
Encouraging family participation	70	(1858)

Figure 8.4   Reported involvement in five health education activities
Source: Latter et al., 1992: 169

England were reported to be involved in these activities as is shown in Figure 8.4.

Only four wards in the country were reported not to have any health education activities at all. These results, from a very large survey, suggest that at a gross level nurses are involved in patient education. The authors acknowledge that perception of activity and actual activity may differ, but even allowing for some over-estimation these results can be taken to support the view that the vast majority of nurses are involved in patient education. There is also evidence to suggest, however, that nurses are not fulfilling their potential in this area of care.

An interesting study was undertaken in an acute care setting by Breemhaar *et al.* (1996) who conducted an ambitious investigation to attempt to determine what information patients desired and what they reported they received, and plotted their route through their hospital admission to identify when and by whom they received information. Thus the study was not specifically relating to information obtained from nurses, rather it was an attempt to capture the entire process of education for inpatients. They included people admitted for herniorraphy (14 patients) or cholecystectomy (20 patients) which are common operations in the Netherlands, where the study took place. The sample size is relatively small but the tracking of each patient through the hospital would have prevented a large-scale study from being feasible. The investigators found that patients experienced fear of anaesthesia and of post-operative pain and reported a lack of information about medical aspects of their disease, the operation, anaesthesia, and discharge. Ambiguity surrounding the roles and responsibilities of the various health care providers they met in hospital was also reported to be a problem.

Patients were found to be exposed to a wide variety of professional groups, an average of 19 for those undergoing herniorraphy and 22 for cholecystectomy patients. There was variability in the amount of information received and the giving of information was found to be largely uncoordinated. They report that physicians, in particular, appeared to be reluctant to respond to patients' inquiries. Patients found they received too much information on admission but too little at discharge. While the sample was gathered in only two hospitals and thus may not be representative of the wider hospital population, the authors report that their findings do not differ too much from other reports on surgical patient education. This lends credibility to their work.

A report such as this may help nurses to develop protocols and to ensure that they play their part in a multi-professional process of patient education. The study could be replicated at a local level to ascertain whether a problem exists in their own locality and, if so, identified factors which could improve the situation can be used to inform the development of protocols, care pathways or evidence-based clinical guidelines. In cases where a large number of people are all contributing a small amount of information it is important that patient education is co-ordinated so that the end result is not fragmented. Nurses are in an ideal position to co-ordinate this activity and as part of a multi-disciplinary team to identify which professionals are responsible for giving which information, at which time and by what means. It is nurses who are the constant presence throughout a patient's experience in hospital, and possibly whilst in the community, and they can then help reinforce or clarify information given by others who may not return to the patient. The authors make the recommendations listed in Figure 8.5 to help improve surgical patient education. All these recommendations sound reasonable and there is scope for nursing to make a contribution to each one of them for the overall improvement of patient education in an acute area.

A similarly fragmented picture of nurse education also emerged from the study by Coonrod et al. (1994) to investigate the proportion of adults with diabetes in America who had received education

---

- the content of information delivered to patients should be improved,
- greater information is required about the roles of different professionals patients are likely to encounter,
- medical aspects of their condition and information about anaesthetics is needed,
- information about behaviour to promote recovery is needed,
- the method of providing information needs to be improved,
- the consistency of information provided needs to be improved,
- information needs to be applied more evenly over the inpatient period,
- unambiguous delineation of the roles and responsibilities of different health care providers is required to ensure neither duplication nor gaps occur in the service provided.

Figure 8.5   Recommendations to help improve education for surgical patients
Source: Bremhaar et al., 1996

about their condition and the source of any such education. They identified that only 35 per cent from a sample of 2405 adults with diabetes had received education in the form of an educational class. However, 97 per cent of the sample had obtained information from some source as is shown in Figure 8.6.

The results of this study demonstrate not only that there are deficiencies in the education process but also that nurses, relative to other professionals, play only a modest part in the process of information-giving. It is important that a strategy is developed to enable patients to be properly educated rather than gleaning knowledge in a piecemeal fashion as is suggested by this study. Nurses have the potential to take a much more proactive role in patient education. They need to state the extent of their responsibility to both colleagues and patients and where they fit into the total patient education process. A systematic approach to education is far more likely to be effective and efficient, as previously cited research has shown. So, although work such as that by Latter *et al.* (1992) indicates that nurses in acute settings are involved in patient education, research such as that by Breemhaar *et al.* (1996) and Coonrod *et al.* (1994) suggests that there is much room for improvement of patient education and that nurses can make a significant contribution to such an improvement.

Source	% patients
Any source	97
Physician in community setting	86
Dietician/nutritionist	28
Physician or nurse in hospital setting	25
Nurse in community setting	18
Relative/friend/other person with diabetes	24
Diabetes education class/organisation	28
Newspaper/library	17
Other	18

Figure 8.6   Sources of information about diabetes
Source: Adapted from Coonrod et al., 1994: 852

Barriers to patient education

A classic analysis of the role of nurses in patient education was presented by Syred in 1981, in an article entitled 'The abdication of the role of health education by hospital nurses'. She suggests that: 'in the ward situation, the nurse appears to abdicate this role, avoiding contact with patients unless performing some specific skill' (Syred, 1981: 27). Almost twenty years later has this situation changed?

The studies cited above, from acute and ongoing illness situations, demonstrate that nurses, while not abdicating their role in patient education, are not playing as full and influential a role in patient education as they could do. It is important to consider why this might be the case. Close (1988) analysed the situation in the late 1980s and concluded that while there is evidence to show that patient education is being done effectively there is also evidence to suggest that it is not done enough. Close identified the following barriers to patient education:

- Lack of knowledge
- Lack of the necessary communication skills
- Lack of assessment skills
- Lack of teaching skills
- Low priority

- The nurse as a source of patient education – both nurses and patients may fail to recognise the nurse as a source of information.

Several of these points relate to a lack of necessary skills and Close (1988) suggests that the problem is attributable to a: 'shortfall in nurse training at basic and post-basic level' (211). This point would be supported by Syred (1981), Tilley *et al.* (1987) and Luker and Caress (1989). However, the picture is more complicated than just a shortfall in nurse education.

Barriers to the process of patient education were also identified by Agre *et al.* (1990) when investigating how much time nurses spend teaching cancer patients. They begin by acknowledging that whilst cancer patients must have information, hospital stays are reduced and there is usually a shortage of nurses. Therefore the educational process must be creative if quality education is to be provided in a cost-effective way. All education given to each patient and his or her family was documented for the duration of 121 patients' hospital stay. In total this represented 825 days of hospitalisation. They report that the average amount of teaching delivered to each patient per day was 16.6 minutes. This was taken to be a significant amount of time and had an associated significant cost. The implications of their study are shown in Figure 8.7.

Problem	Nursing shortage
	Patients spend less time in hospital
Leading to	Less time for patient education
Possible solutions	The need to supplement one-to-one teaching
Avenues to explore	Closed circuit television
	Written educational material
	Group classes
Evaluation	Comparisons of time it takes to teach specific information using different methods

Figure 8.7 Nursing implications for patient teaching
Source: Agre *et al.*, 1990: 38

When discussing some of the barriers to patient education Agre *et al.* acknowledge that not all solutions are in the hands of practitioners but that managerial support in also required:

> No one would argue that for professional, moral, ethical and legal reasons nurses should be teaching. But is it reasonable that in today's climate of high costs for patient care, hospitals and especially nursing departments should be expected to absorb the cost of teaching . . . send patients home earlier and more safely.
>
> (Agre *et al.*, 1990: 38)

In contrast to the study by Agre *et al.*, Honan *et al.* (1988) report that many nurses (54 out of 60 (90 per cent)) did not think they had sufficient time to teach. The great majority of the nurses in their study (47 (78 per cent)) responded that they spent more time doing informal rather than formal teaching. Only 2 nurses (3 per cent) reported that they spent the majority of their time doing formal education while 9 (15 per cent) reported that they spent equal amounts of time on formal and informal teaching. Overall the study found that factors which promoted patient education included acknowledged responsibility for teaching, giving the activity high priority over other aspects of care and knowledge. Lack of materials, unsuitable environment, too little time and poor staffing levels were reported to be interfering factors.

Other factors have also been cited as barriers to patient education, such as lack of confidence to teach (Price, 1985); lack of resources (Bird *et al.*, 1994); lack of control over the patients' stay in hospital undermining the ability to plan ahead (Luker and Caress, 1989); nurses being too busy with routines and rituals for which they have no rationale to be able to devote time to patient education (Walsh and Ford, 1989); nurses choosing to distance themselves from close but potentially stressful relationships with patients (Menzies, 1960) although this may be required to help reduce anxiety in patients (Swindale, 1989) or involved in chronic illness situations (Dunn, 1995; Sleight, 1995).

These are all important points and should not be overlooked if nurses are to improve their contribution to patient education. As patient education is an important part of care and also a vital component of nursing if holistic care is to be delivered, rather than relegate patient education to another 'nice but extra' part of the service, it is important to consider whether any steps can be made to facilitate patient education by nurses.

Facilitating patient education

Literature suggests there are several ways in which successful patient education could be facilitated and the main ones are mentioned below.

Deciding the scope of practice in relation to patient education

All qualified nurses have a role to play in patient education which is a legitimate area of nursing endeavour. In addition to the reasons given at the beginning of this chapter it is believed that politically it is important that nurses defend their role in patient education, because other professional groups, who may be no more able to do it than nurses, will readily take over this function and an important aspect of nursing practice could be written out of job descriptions. However, it is also vital that nurses raise their standards and undertake patient education that can be defended by research whenever possible and can be demonstrated to have an impact upon patient care. Only then will it be endorsed and supported at managerial and policy making levels. Ill-defined, randomly offered, unplanned or unstructured patient education is not a sufficient approach to practice in the current health care climate. Nurses could not be involved in other aspects of care, for example lifting and handling of patients, without first defining their remit, identifying the resources they need and the way in which important information will be documented, yet evidence suggests that a considerable amount, but by no means all, of patient education is conducted without the benefit of much forward planning.

A possible way forward is for nurses, or nurses as part of the health care team, at ward, community or locality levels to identify the educational needs of the main categories of patients in their care. This is not to suggest a standardised approach to all types of patient, far from it, but there are likely to be common trends in educational provision in different types of care such as in casualty, intensive care, acute surgery or rehabilitation settings. Nurses could then define what they believe to be an appropriate scope of practice for nurses in this area of practice. What are patients likely to need, what is it reasonable for nurses to aim to provide?

It may be feasible to identify a continuum of interventions, from most simple through to the more complicated requirements, as described previously (see Figure 8.3) and relate this to levels of patient education. From this information nurses should be able to clarify which aspects of patient education all qualified nurses can participate in; for example, to undertake an initial assessment of learning needs (for patients with complex needs it may then be appropriate for more advanced level practitioners to be involved), provide information, document patient education, liaise with other health professionals and co-ordinate educational input to ensure that patients do receive appropriate education. All nurses should be able to participate in planning the form of patient education to be given in their area, whether it will be one-to-one or group teaching, whether information leaflets will be used and if so which ones are most appropriate. If educational aids are to be used, the nurses need to be aware of what they cover and where the equipment is stored. As educational aids should be a supplement to, rather than a substitute for, direct communication, nurses must decide on appropriate follow-up for patients after watching a video or using a computer-based package in order to clarify issues which patients may raise.

It is at this stage that specialist nurses can have an important part to play. They can play a leading role in identifying needs and helping to plan and structure appropriate teaching interventions for particular groups of patients. While they alone may not be responsible for the delivery of all education they can be instrumental in developing teaching interventions and help clarify which level of nurse can undertake which aspects of patient education. Nurse specialists would be expected to have a greater knowledge of research and resources relevant to their particular area and they can help disseminate this information to others. Luker and Kendrick (1995) present an interesting study along these lines when they illustrate how the results of a large volume of research was synthesised by specialist nurses, points for good practice were decided upon and then disseminated for use by district nurses. This method of intervention was found to be a helpful way of promoting evidence-based practice and could be applied to other areas.

While much of this may sound like common sense, from the results of some of the studies presented in this book it seems quite likely that in many clinical settings ongoing patient education occurs as a result of tradition and availability. Perhaps medical representatives from pharmaceutical companies have left literature or videos so they are used because they are to hand, or leaflets are given out because they are available, without appraising their suitability for a particular client group. Patients deemed to need reassurance will often have *'provide reassurance'* written in their care plan without any prior analysis of what is required to reduce anxiety in a particular situation, thus the activity becomes a cliché rather than a valuable intervention. As patient education is very rarely evaluated little is known about the effect that such interventions may have.

Only after deciding on the scope of practice relating to patient education will it be possible to look ahead realistically and to clarify other issues such as organisational factors, recourses, time and preparation of staff.

Organisational issues which influence the success of patient education

An important organisational issue appears to be the need to plan realistically and aim to conduct patient education within the confines of existing services. Patient education programmes or interventions which require changes to other aspects of the service which are thought to work well are unlikely to succeed. This point was noted by Jenny (1990) when reporting examples of exemplary patient education programmes available in Canada, which includes the work in the Shaughnessay Hospital, Vancouver, in which an extensive but simple patient education programme was developed over an eight-year period. She notes that it was designed to: '. . . fit so snugly into the routines of patient care that it would become as accepted and familiar a part of the care as routine vital signs' (Durbach, 1986, cited by Jenny, 1990).

Breemhaar *et al.* (1996) also stress that for a programme to be effective it must be designed to integrate well with other aspects of care:

> successful implementation of patient education measures which are suited for application by hospital staff members, requires their compatibility with everyday hospital practices and with skills and attitudes of hospital staff members. This is required first because regular treatment and care tasks should not be disrupted by patient education measures.

(32)

Thus it is important to aim from the outset for a realistic form of patient education which is compatible and integrated into routine care. However, this does not mean that no changes should be made or that extra interventions cannot be 'slotted in' to the existing scheme of practice. As was noted in Chapter 4, several authors reported success when teaching patients prior to admission to hospital (Scriven and Tucker, 1997; Theis and Johnson, 1995), thus a successful intervention was added in without upsetting existing schedules of events.

Ruzicki (1989) advocated the need to plan ahead, to standardise interventions where possible, to design educational programmes to suit groups of patients likely to be encountered. Such planning will serve to save time in the long term. Clearly individual assessment is still required as programmes will be modified according to individualised need. But there is unlikely to be a need to design each patient's educational programme from scratch in every case. It is, of course, equally unlikely that any two patients will benefit from identical, standardised, pre-prescribed educational interventions with no allowance made for individual needs and differences.

Another factor to consider is the way in which nursing care itself is organised. The work of Thomas (1994) has suggested that nursing organised on a primary nursing basis may facilitate verbal interaction with patients, improve the explanations given, and help staff to know their patients better than on team or task nursing wards. They report that these findings held, regardless of whether it was a nursing auxiliary or a qualified nurse who was being observed. Thus the extra patient contact afforded by primary nursing may offer better opportunities for patients and nurses to engage in education than in other forms of organisation. While primary nursing is still not widely practised in hospital settings it is worth noting that this method of organising care may help improve patient education.

As a result of the study by Honan et al. (1988) to 'describe registered nurses' perceptions of their responsibilities in patient teaching' (33) the authors made ten recommendations to enable patient education to be enhanced. Only one of these relates to improving staff teaching ability, the rest relate to organisational issues. The recommendations are illustrated in Figure 8.8.

The work of other researchers in this area would also support the need for managerial support if nurses are to have a successful role in patient education, for example, Latter et al. (1992) and Luker and Caress (1989).

1   use a multidisciplinary approach for patient teaching programmes;
2   conduct classes covering specific clinical knowledge areas;
3   provide in-services on teaching/learning techniques;
4   develop inclusive guidance teaching sheets with an improved documentation system;
5   provide an environment conducive to patient teaching;
6   designate a central area for patient-teaching materials on all units;
7   incorporate a patient-teaching co-ordinator in health institutions;
8   implement a documentation system to determine with certainty whether or not a patient has been taught;
9   provide more time and staff;
10   integrate into basic nursing programmes the role of educator and teaching/learning techniques.

Figure 8.8 Registered nurses' perceptions of their responsibilities in patient teaching
Source: Modified from Honan *et al.*, 1988: 37

Justifying the time spent on patient education

A reported barrier to patient education was lack of time. This is a commonly cited reason for all sorts of short-comings in nursing care. Lack of time should not automatically be used as a reason to delegate patient education to other professionals (who are also short of time). The suggested need for more time for patient teaching also provides an opportunity to evaluate critically the way in which nurses use their time. Perhaps they spend time on activities which should not be given preferential priority over patient education. For example, Busby and Gilchrist (1992) investigated the nurses' role when on ward rounds and concluded that this activity may not be a good use of nursing time. Yet, how often do nurses prioritise teaching patients over attending ward rounds? Similarly, Webb (1995: 919) presented an interesting list of examples of non-nursing activities pursued by theatre nurses at the expense of patient education:

•   Restocking rooms with supplies
•   Ordering and putting away stores

- Acting as a messenger for surgeons etc.
- Answering bleeps and telephones
- Fetching and carrying non-urgent equipment, trolleys etc.
- Preparation of operating room furniture before the start of operating lists
- Clearing away and cleaning trolleys and equipment after each case and at the end of each list

Walsh and Ford (1989) illustrate very well that once we critically examine the way nurses spend time there is usually evidence to suggest that many activities are not as central to the nursing function as is often believed. However, patient education is an activity which we could defend as being vital both for patients and nurses and requiring a higher priority on the nursing agenda than is often the case at present.

The need for more time to teach patients could be used as leverage to negotiate for more staff *if* it could be demonstrated that patient education, when delivered by nurses, was effective and efficient. It is, however, impossible to defend the need for patient education or the staff to do it if there is no demonstrable outcome from the resources invested in it.

It should also be noted that providing more time and staff to undertake patient education may not, in the long term, be an expensive option. For example, when the annual cost of non-insulin-dependent diabetes to the National Health Service was calculated it was estimated to be £5 billion for direct costs (King's Fund, 1996). This analysis does not include indirect costs such as days off work. Thus the total costs to the nation are even higher. The majority of the money is spent on treatment of the chronic complications of the disease, many of which can be reduced, delayed or even avoided with appropriate self-management, a prerequisite for which is patient education. Greater amounts of money invested in patient education now could well reduce the costs of diabetes in the future. The same could be true of other conditions, as is suggested by Sleight (1995) with reference to people with hypertension:

> Teaching communication skills is arguably *the* most important part of medical education, not an optional extra. . . . Overall, communication and rapport with the patient and his family are of prime importance in the prevention of the consequences of high blood pressure. People die not from pressure alone, but

from the effects of that pressure on their arteries, so many other factors come into the equation. Building customer loyalty in hypertension needs all the skills we can muster, both for treatment and more importantly for prevention.

(Sleight, 1995: 69)

Clearly, we would need to be able to demonstrate that patient education can lead to reduced expenditure. To some extent this has been achieved through the work of Bartlett (1995) who conducted a cost-benefit analysis of patient education. He found that amongst the studies consulted, none reported that the education cost more than it saved and frequently, but not always, education could lead to significant savings. The results of his analysis 'support the notion that efforts to reduce the demand for healthcare services not only can save costs but they can also improve quality outcomes' (90). Consequently, he made important recommendations aimed at policy makers and administrators in recognition that the context in which patient education occurs is vital to the success of the operation. The recommendations are illustrated in Figure 8.9.

This analysis helps defend the use of time and resources for patient teaching, it is an example to nurses of how we must be able to also justify the use of time and finally this work serves to demonstrate that nurses alone cannot solve all problems relating to patient education. There must be support at all levels not just at the actual

---

1   Assure that patient education is supported through national policy and/or legislation.

2   Integrate patient education into practice guidelines and critical care pathways.

3   Include patients/consumers in making assessments of quality of care.

4   Revise institutional accreditation criteria to include patient education (presumably relating to America).

5   Recognise the tendency for urgent medical care services to dominate funding requests. Assure a proper balance of funding between preventative and therapeutic services.

Figure 8.9   Recommendations for policy relating to improving patient education

Source: Bartlett, 1995: 90

delivery of the care. This point was also emphasised by Visser (1996) who noted that successful patient education could not be the responsibility of any single profession, rather it had to be a concerted effort amongst a range of professionals:

> The development of patient education and counseling is based on the co-operation of several actors: patients, providers, policy makers, researchers and authors. Each of these actors have their own rights and duties as well as their view on the contribution of the other parties.
>
> (Visser, 1996: 1)

The need for suitable preparation to be a patient educator

Once the nature and scope of patient education has been agreed upon the preparation of nurses to be involved in it can be undertaken in a more focused manner. When considering barriers to successful patient education one of the recurring themes was inadequate preparation to enable nurses to undertake the role.

A good knowledge base including the topics to be taught and an understanding of the teaching process is clearly vital if nurses are to be effective educators. Luker and Caress (1989) present a strong argument that nurses in general do not have the necessary knowledge base from which to conduct successful patient education. Consequently they state that it would not be wise, realistic or desirable for all nurses to be involved in patient education as it is such a complex process. They argue that the breadth and depth of knowledge required by nurses on general wards or in community settings who encounter patients with a wide variety of clinical conditions places unrealistic expectations on nurses. Rather than advocate that nurses in general are suitably prepared, Luker and Caress support the idea of specialist nurses having a greater part to play in patient education and play down the role of general nurses. This is not the approach advocated in this chapter, as has already been explained. However, the more complex forms of educational interventions such as that suggested by Dunn (1995) do need greater levels of expertise and knowledge than could be expected of more junior members of nursing staff. Education which depends on the formation of ongoing relationships and is aimed at promoting empowerment, or equality of power, will need greater educational preparation than is usually available to nurses on pre-registration courses; such educational input will require professionals with highly developed teaching skills.

The following extracts from the work of Stewart Dunn support this perspective.

> The human relationship between professional and patient is the cornerstone of long-term management in chronic illness. It is both perilous and unprofessional to ignore the human factor on either side of the consulting room since health care providers are motivated by precisely the same human instincts as are their patients.
>
> (Dunn, 1995: 134)

> Ultimately, professional training for chronic illness must shift towards a focus on the long-term benefits of the continuing relationship between patient and provider and the broader health care team.
>
> (ibid.: 136)

So how do we teach nurses to improve their knowledge of the subjects to be taught, communication skills and the teaching process? In the literature there are examples of techniques to help health professionals improve their educational skills (Faulkner, 1993; Faulkner, 1994; Maguire et al., 1978). While having a good grasp of the material to be taught and of the appropriate skills to undertake patient education is vital, the philosophical perspective from which nurses will endeavour to plan their work in education is also essential (Caraher, 1998; Coates and Boore, 1995; Caraher, 1994). To help them to move away from an authoritarian educational model nurses will need to be prepared to be involved in levels of patient teaching which are more complex than simply giving information (Feste and Anderson, 1995).

It is equally important to recognise that weaknesses in education competencies are not restricted to nurses; all health professionals require appropriate preparation. Therefore whoever is elected to undertake complicated patient education will need to be prepared for the role and a financial investment made to help promote their skills (Sleight, 1995).

Jenny (1990) made an interesting point when considering exemplary practice at the Shaughnessay Hospital, referred to earlier, when she noted that: 'Patient education is a major component of new staff nurses' orientation to the hospital and their patient teaching ability is assessed in the annual performance appraisal of staff nurses' (51).

How often is this the case in other hospitals? Yet if patient education is to be a valued activity in nursing why should this form of recognition not be made?

Evidence-based patient education

Politically it is important that nurses stake their claim in patient education and prove that they are able to do it and do it well. In Chapter 2 the importance of evidence-based practice for nurses involved in patient education was discussed and will be briefly revisited in this chapter.

It is now over a quarter of a century since the Briggs committee (HMSO, 1972) urged nursing to become a research-based profession yet according to recent reports, using research as a basis for nursing practice remains a problem (Camiah, 1997; Webb and Mackenzie, 1993; Clifford, 1993; Bircumshaw, 1990; Hunt, 1987). In the case of patient education nurses clearly have a long way to go if practice is to be research-based. In the course of this book a wealth of material relating to research and patient education has been presented. However, the vast majority of practising nurses are probably unaware of much of the research available to support patient education in their own area of practice. Many attempts to understand the reasons why nurses tend not to use research as a basis for practice have been made. Dunn *et al.* (1998) investigated reported barriers to using research in practice amongst a convenience sample of 316 nurses working in the United Kingdom. Figure 8.10 illustrates the top 10 barriers as reported by nurses in the UK and are compared with the results when the BARRIERS Scale (Funk *et al.*, 1991) was applied in America.

This is an interesting study and the results support those of other research in this area. The implications of these perceived barriers are helpful when aiming to promote the utilisation of research in practice. All of these points are potentially relevant to research in patient education. As was noted in the section 'Facilitating patient education', Figure 8.10 demonstrates that factors such as setting, and presentation of research as well as those directly relating to nurses affect the uptake of research. Thus using research is not the sole responsibility of nurses. Nurses cannot be expected to make

Factor	Item	% rating*	
		UK	USA
Setting	There is insufficient time on the job to implement new ideas	75	75
Setting	Physicians will not co-operate with implementation	72	71
Setting	Facilities are inadequate for implementation	68	68
Setting	Nurse does not have time to read research	67	67
Presentation	Statistical analyses not understandable	75	68
Presentation	Relevant literature not compiled in one place	70	63
Presentation	Research not reported clearly and readably	67	54
Nursing	Nurse does not feel capable of evaluating the quality of research	70	59
Nursing	Nurse is unaware of the research	67	74
No specific factor	The amount of research information is overwhelming	66	not reported

* % rating item as great or moderate barrier
Figures rounded to whole numbers

Figure 8.10   Top 10 barriers to using research in the UK and USA
Source: Adapted from Dunn et al., 1998: 1207

use of research findings on their own – it has to be a team effort. The team must involve researchers, who should present their work in a user-friendly way; nurse-teachers who must help nurses get to grips with reading research reports and the process of conducting research (Clifford, 1993); specialist nurses, who have an important part to play as they can help translate results into implications for practice in a relevant way (Lacey, 1994); and administrators and managers who must provide tangible support and encouragement for research implementation which will improve patient care. All these factors are important, as well as the actions of practising nurses, who with appropriate back-up must be willing to base practice on evidence when possible.

Lacey (1994) found in her study to investigate research utilisation in nursing practice that a major difficulty cited by many respondents was a lack of resources, if using the research would involve expense. Nurses on their own cannot provide financial investment in the implementation of research. They require appropriate support from managers and administrators. However, nurses do have to justify to such people why they believe the research is worthwhile. As has already been pointed out in this chapter some financial investment will be required to help promote the use of research in practice, but this must then lead to improved quality of care and possibly the chance to save money in the future. Nurses may be expected to develop an argument to defend investing money to help promote research-based practice. The support of professionals in other health care disciplines is required as nurses do not work alone. In particular, the support of doctors has been found to be essential (Morris, 1998; Lacey, 1994).

All these people are necessary in addition to practising nurses, who with appropriate back-up must be motivated to base practice on evidence when possible. An important finding reported by Lacey (1994) was that:

> Nurses are generally favourable towards research, and are willing to implement it when they feel able to and are confident of findings.
>
> (994)

This is a positive finding and such an attitude needs to be fostered and developed. If nurses' attempts to implement research are constantly frustrated then the goal of evidence-based practice will become even more remote.

The need for nurses to work collaboratively to promote research use is supported by Goode et al. (1987) (in Lacey, 1994) who stated that:

> The success of research utilization depends on organizational co-operation, as well as the skills and motivation of nursing staff members. Nursing in clinical settings needs a practical

systematic approach to the process of research utilization. Only then can we hope to effect research driven change to our practice.

(988)

The work of Camiah (1997) presents a useful model by which research can be applied in practice using a team approach including researchers, nursing lecturers and practitioners to work together to facilitate and promote research in practice. Too often using research is not seen as a collaborative multi-professional activity.

Alison Tierney (1993: 386) warns nurses of the urgent need to be able to 'justify the costs of preferred interventions and systems of care delivery' if nursing is to survive in the current market economy. As has been advocated throughout this book, as far as is possible nurses must strive to demonstrate that patient education is a valuable intervention which can make an impact on patient care and on patient quality of life if it is to be supported by health care commissioners in the future. As Buchan (1992) (cited by Tierney, 1993: 386) has pointed out:

> At a time of cost containment the real challenge for all nurses is to ensure that it is cost-effectiveness not cost-cutting on the managerial agenda. . . . If nurses ignore this issue, important decisions on resource allocation will be made by administrators with a strong knowledge of costing but a weaker appreciation of the impact of cost-containment strategies on the quality of nursing care.

Thus there is a need for nurses to be aware of research material relevant to their own area of practice, and with facilities such as computer-based literature searches this is not such an arduous task as it once was. Nurses must be prepared to make use of relevant findings when they are available and with appropriate support strive to apply research in practice. Finally, nurses must be involved in evaluating the impact of their teaching if they are to demonstrate that their interventions are worthwhile. Again they cannot undertake this work on their own but they do need to accept that they can contribute to the research effort in nursing as it is vital that research is closely linked to practice. As Kappeli (1993) has pointed out, practising nurses have a vital role to play in the research process and the development of knowledge relevant to nursing care. It is by reflecting on practice, being aware of research and using it, and if necessary criticising it, that nurses can help advance nursing practice. As such nurses have a vital role to play and must not assume advancing professional care can be left to others.

Having said all this it must be noted that the research base for patient education is far from complete. As Herbert (1996) has noted: 'Yet our knowledge of how best to provide information to people to allow informed decision making and to enhance retention of information is still very incomplete' (121).

The review in Chapter 2 also illustrated that not all research is good enough to use. There are still many gaps in our knowledge, it would be wrong to imply that there is an answer to all our questions about patient education. There is a wealth of research material available to inform nursing practice; however there is still work to be done. Redman (1993) has also commented that a lot of work on patient education is still required. She reviewed the progress made in patient education over the past 25 years and concluded that while there had been slow advancement there was still basic developmental work remaining to be done. She listed the following eight points as areas which she believes need to be considered:

1 *There is really no adequate description of learning conditions under which education for patients takes place.*

This is a fundamental issue. A variety of theories about learning have been included in this book and the relevance to patients rather than fit, healthy adults has been discussed. There is still much to be understood about how learning takes place when people are ill and anxious. We have yet to identify when is the best time for people to learn, how we can motivate them to be self-caring or to undertake long-term behavioural change.

2 *There is no standardised way of describing teaching interventions, and in some literature they are not described in any detail at all and thus the studies could not be replicated.*

This point was discussed in Chapter 2 when problems and weaknesses in studies reporting teaching interventions were discussed in detail.

3 *It would be useful to conceptualise patient education services on a continuum from knowledge development to complex behaviour change.*

This point was also discussed in this chapter and the work of Dunn (1995) presented to illustrate this issue. A tentative continuum was presented in Figure 8.7 to form the basis for further work. However, as was stated before, this type of schedule is important as it will help to identify the broad spectrum of patient education and the associated range of skills, resources and interventions required to facilitate the education of patients with differing educational needs.

> 4 *There is no organised pressure group to focus on direction for development of the field and on assurance of workplace conditions that support patient education.*

This is a very important point as without influential support at policy-making and managerial levels, the future of patient education may not be adequately represented and promoted. Nurses' professional groups, such as within the Royal College of Nursing, are one way in which pressure at political levels can be applied. In America there is some evidence of nationally set standards for patient education programmes, such as for people with asthma (Sheffer and Taggart, 1993) or in diabetes (Clement, 1995). These are important pressure groups, they will help to improve educational standards, although they are not spear-headed by nurses. On the whole, lobbying and policy-making at a national level is a rather under-developed aspect of nursing (Clay, 1987). Traditionally nurses have not been good at actively developing the profession. Years of dominance by the medical profession has led to nurses feeling relatively disempowered. The current need to run the National Health Service like a business which must be effective and efficient may make nurses feel even less powerful.

As Kappeli (1993) points out, too often patients and nurses find themselves at the bottom of the institutional hierarchy. She argues that in a general sense nurses must define their professional role more clearly and have greater sway in influencing policy which affects care. This point is also highly pertinent to the development of nurses in patient education:

> clinical nurses themselves must learn to assert themselves as professionals on behalf of their patients and stop doing everything for everybody. They must learn to perceive their task as distinct from that of cleaners, housekeepers and kitchen staff without feeling guilty in discriminating between them. . . . They

need the power to influence structures, environment and other professional groups according to the needs of direct care.

(Kappeli, 1993: 209)

5 *Technology should be much more imaginatively used. The potential for computers to enhance the teaching/learning process is apparently occurring only very slowly.*

This issue was discussed in Chapter 5 and is largely self-explanatory. However, as the population at large becomes increasingly computer literate the use of technology in patient education will also advance. Serious development of telemedicine and telematics is currently underway at international levels and whilst at pilot stages at the present will play a major role in patient support in years to come.

6 *Besides a shift to learning theory that is patient-centred some observers believe that, in the face of competition, health care institutions and practitioners will shift their practice and services to meet needs of customers.*

Redman (1993) notes that conventional treatment has tended to behave 'as if caring for such human needs is beyond its purpose' (28). However, in response to increasing chronic illness she suggests that much greater measures to promote patient self-care and self-management will be called for. She notes also, that patients can only be active participants in their care and contribute to decision making if they are informed and knowledgeable about their options and their condition: 'Truly, such a system would require individualized patient education reaching goals to the patients' satisfaction and integrated with all care, as opposed to being an appendage delivered when time and resources might allow' (728). An interesting thought!

7 *Consideration of the ethics of patient education should undergo rapid evolution.*

Recognising that until the late 1960s health care professionals tended to decide what information the patients needed to know Redman (1993) suggests that information was dispensed to patients if the professionals felt it would be good for them. These days patients are much more likely to be viewed as entitled to the whole truth. However, Redman believes that if patients are to be able to be maximally involved in decision making there are ethical components to this aspiration. Informed consent is viewed as the simplest and a minimal involvement while the problems of making decisions in the face of uncertainty and of choosing health care interventions of limited predictability are seen as issues which embrace moral and ethical issues to which we have not, as yet, given much thought.

> 8 *Healthcare systems worldwide are undergoing reform, so it is important that nursing has a voice in these reforms.*

This point reiterates that of number 4 and is stressing the need for nurses to ensure they have an influential part to play when health care policy for the future is being decided upon.

Conclusion to chapter

In this chapter a case has been made that traditionally, nurses, for all sorts of reasons, have had a role to play in patient education. It is important that nursing continues to play a central role in this aspect of patient care. However, in the current health care climate of very rapid turnover of patients both at inpatient level and in community settings, it can be very difficult to engage in effective, efficient patient education. Factors which have been found to adversely affect patient education were noted and possible ways to encourage and ease the way in which patients can be educated were discussed. Finally, the need to base practice on research has never been greater and some of the difficulties in using research in practice were reviewed. Many articles have been written about the need for nurses to use research but the case is made in this chapter that nurses involved in patient care on a daily basis cannot, single-handedly, improve standards of patient education, base education on research or evaluate teaching programmes and quality of care. All these jobs must be done but not by nurses on their own. The environment has to be conducive to patient education and for this to happen a multi-professional approach is required. While nurses can be key players in the educational process with patients they will need the support of at least, policy makers, managers and administrators, medical colleagues and other nurses. In return nurses must aim to demonstrate that resources invested in patient education can make a difference to patient care.

KEY POINTS FROM CHAPTER 8

1 *Nurses as educators of patients*: throughout this chapter it is argued that nurses must be involved in patient education, that they must bring their unique combinations of knowledge relating to health, illness and disease; patient education; interpersonal communication skills; holistic approaches to patient care; and their central role in coordinating and managing patient care, together to enhance the practice and outcomes of patient education overall.

2 *Nurses need to clarify their role in patient education.* Only through a more focused understanding of what nurses are aiming to achieve can appropriate interventions be planned and developed. Greater clarification of role will help nurses to identify the resources they need and the specific education required to enable them to deliver it. Research suggests that such moves will foster effectiveness and efficiency in patient education.

3 *Research indicates that nurses have not yet reached their full potential* in patient education and concurrently evidence has confirmed that patients' educational needs are not adequately met. In addition to which, it has also been shown that only a small amount of patients' knowledge is gained from nurses. There is surely room for nurses to develop their expertise in this aspect of care and in so doing strive to more fully meet the educational needs of patients.

4 *Organisational issues have a great impact on the work of nurses* and it is stressed that nurses cannot improve the standard of patient education in a vacuum. The context in which care is delivered, such as staffing levels, skill mix, prioritising of different aspects of care, provision of resources and support of other members of the health care team for example will all have an effect upon the quality of patient education delivered by nurses.

5 *To help improve the standard of educational practice there have been calls for this aspect of care to be supported through national policy or legislation.* By leaving patient education at an informal level its importance is undermined. For example, nurses can teach if they choose to do so and if they have time and are able. Unfortunately, there is no imperative to provide

patient education with the current levels of policy and standards set at national level.

6 *Nurses need to be suitably prepared to provide effective patient education*. A good knowledge of the topics to be taught, an understanding of the teaching process and good interpersonal communication skills are required for information-giving, which is considered the simplest form of patient education (misleadingly simple in fact). Education which aims to alter attitudes and behaviour is even more difficult to deliver effectively, therefore, nurses involved in this form of patient education must be suitably prepared. As a profession we are not allowed to proceed with other aspects of care, for example giving medications, moving and handling, without appropriate preparation, so why should patient education be treated differently if it is to be valued as an important activity?

7 *Nurses must be able to justify the time and resources* required to undertake patient education effectively. Therefore they must evaluate the outcomes of educational activity and demonstrate that it makes a difference. Otherwise those managing and funding the service will not be convinced of the need to invest in this aspect of patient care.

8 *Evidence-based patient education* – politically it is important that nurses stake their claim in patient education and prove that they are able to do it and to do it well. Wherever possible nurses should base practice on research evidence. Thus nurses must be aware of research relevant to their own area of practice. It is not up to nurses on their own to put research into practice as this must be a team effort but it is reasonable to expect nurses to be aware of research relevant to patient education in their own clinical area.

9 *Drawing from the analysis of Redman (1993)* eight key points which need to be addressed in the future to facilitate the development of patient education are discussed.

CONCLUDING REMARKS – THE BOOK AS
A WHOLE

Looking back over this book, we began by considering the need for patient education and selection of an appropriate definition to help provide a focus for the study, the definition being:

> planned combinations of learning activities designed to assist people who are having or have had experience with illness or disease in making changes in their behaviour conducive to health.
>
> (Squyres, 1980: 1, after Green et al., 1979)

Key issues within the definition were examined during the course of this book. Each chapter was designed to help this definition to be translated into practice. In Chapter 1 the aim was to set the scene for the remainder of the book. As learning does not take place in isolation from other aspects of care and the rest of an individual's life, material to help place patient education into a broad context was presented. Chapter 2 concerned the need to consider the research basis for patient education most carefully, warning that not all that is published is credible. Points to help identify valid research were raised. Only through access to valid research results is it possible to plan combinations of learning activities which have some scientific basis. It may be assumed that successfully to *plan appropriate combinations of learning activities* an understanding of the way people learn and may be influenced to change behaviour conducive to their overall health would be an advantage. Therefore in Chapter 3 theories to help us understand how people learn cognitive material and in Chapter 6, theories to explain how people may change health behaviour, were presented and discussed. Although there are limitations with the application of current educational theories to health care situations it would be unfortunate if we abandoned the use of any theory to guide practice. There remains a need for both theory and practice to be developed, tested and modified until we can claim to understand how people with an illness or disease learn. Only then can we plan educational interventions with an underlying theoretical framework. However, the activities of theory and practice development are closely interlinked and interdependent and while theory is important it cannot be developed without it being tested in practice. In order to deliver planned educational activities there must be a means of organising the work and in Chapters 4 and 5 a process of patient education is examined. Starting with assessment of educational need, identification of problems and setting goals, through selection and delivery of educational interventions to, finally, the evaluation of patient education, all aspects of the process are considered. Research-based evidence to help provide a scientific foundation for practice was included throughout Chapters 4 and 5. Educational interventions with both affective and cognitive dimensions are the focus of Chapter 7. They can involve all that was discussed in Chapters 4 and 5 but are complicated by the intention to change behaviour, not just increase cognitive knowledge (although this is no mean feat in itself). Finally, in Chapter 8 the involvement of nurses in patient education was considered. Factors which help this activity and those which hinder it were discussed and priorities for patient education development in the future were identified.

References

Abley, C. (1997) Teaching elderly patients how to use inhalers. A study to evaluate an educational programme on inhaler technique, for elderly patients, *Journal of Advanced Nursing*, 25: 699–708.

Agre, P., Bookbinder, M., Cirrincione, C. and Keating, E. (1990) How much time do nurses spend teaching cancer patients?, *Patient Education and Counseling*, 16: 29–38.

Agre, P., Kurtz, R.C. and Krauss, B.J. (1994) A randomized trial using videotape to present consent information for colonoscopy, *Gastrointestinal Endoscopy*, 40(3): 271–276.

Ajzen, I. (1988) *Attitudes, Personality and Behaviour*, Milton Keynes: Open University Press.

Albert, T. and Chadwick, S. (1992) How readable are practice leaflets?, *British Medical Journal*, 305: 1266–1268.

Allen, J.D. and Hall, B.A. (1988) Challenging the focus on technology: a critique of the medical model in a changing health care system, *Advances in Nursing Science*, 10 (3): 22–34.

Anderson, L.A. and Sharpe, P.A. (1991) Improving patient and provider communication: a synthesis and review of communication intervention, *Patient Education and Counseling*, 17: 99–134.

Anderson, R.A., Funnell, M.M., Butler, P.M., Arnold, M.S., Fitzgerald, J.T. and Feste, C.C. (1995) Patient empowerment: results of a randomized controlled trial, *Diabetes Care*, 18(7): 943–949.

Anderson, R.M. (1986) The personal meaning of having diabetes: implications for patient behaviour and education or kicking the bucket theory, *Diabetic Medicine*, 3: 85–89.

Anderson, R.M. (1995) Patient empowerment and the traditional medical model: a case of irreconcilable differences?, *Diabetes Care*, 18(3): 412–415.

Anderson, R.M., Fitzgerald, J.T., Gorenflo, D.W. and Oh, M.S. (1993) A comparison of the diabetes-related attitudes of health care professionals and patients, *Patient Education and Counseling*, 21: 41–50.

Antrobus, S. (1997) An analysis of nursing in context: the effects of current health policy, *Journal of Advanced Nursing*, 25: 447–453.

Arborelius, E. and Osterberg, E. (1995) How do GPs discuss subjects other than illness?, *Patient Education and Counseling*, 25: 257–268.

Arthur, V.A.M. (1995) Written patient information: a review of the literature, *Journal of Advanced Nursing*, 21: 1081–1086.

Ashworth, P.D., Longmate, M.A. and Morrison, P. (1992) Patient participation: its meaning and significance in the context of caring, *Journal of Advanced Nursing* 17: 1430–1439.

Assal, J.-Ph., Berger, M., Gay, N. and Canivet, J. (1983) *Diabetes Education: How to Improve Patient Education*, Amsterdam, Oxford and Princeton: Excerpta Medica.

Audit Commission (1993) *What Seems to be the Matter: Communication Between Hospitals and Patients*, London: HMSO.

Ausubel, D.P., Novak, J.D. and Hanesian, H. (1978) *Educational Psychology: A Cognitive View*, 2nd edition, New York: Holt, Rinehart and Winston.

Avis, M. (1994) Choice cuts; an exploratory study of patients' views about participation in decision-making in a day surgery unit, *International Journal of Nursing Studies* 31(3): 289–298.

Baggott, R. (1994) Health and Health Care in Britain, London: The Macmillan Press Ltd.

Bandura, A. (1977a) Self-efficacy: toward a unifying theory of behavioural change, *Psychological Review*, 84: 191–215.

Bandura, A. (1977b) *Social Learning Theory*, Englewood Cliffs, NJ: Prentice Hall.

Bandura, A. (1986) *Social Foundations of Thought and Action: A Social Cognitive Theory*, Englewood, NJ: Prentice-Hall.

Barber, J.H., McEwan, C. and Yates, B.D. (1995) Video, health education and the General Practitioner Contract, *Health Bulletin*, 53(5): 326–333.

Barnum, B.J.S. (1990) *Nursing Theory. Analysis, Application, Evaluation*, 3rd edition, Glenview, IL: Scott, Foresman/Little, Brown Higher Education.

Bartlett, E.E. (1989) Patient education can lower costs, improve quality, *Hospitals*, 5 November: 88.

Bartlett, E.E. (1990) The telephone: an under-exploited patient education vehicle, *Patient Education and Counseling*, 15: 215–216.

Bartlett, E.E. (1995) Cost-benefit analysis of patient education, *Patient Education and Counseling*, 26: 87–91.

Bartlett, E.E., Grayson, M., Barker, R., Levine, D.M., Golden, A. and Libber, S. (1984) The effects of physician communications skills on patient satisfaction: recall, and adherence, *Journal of Chronic Disease*, 37(9/10): 755–764.

Basler, H. (1995) Patient education with reference to the process of behavioural change, *Patient Education and Counseling*, 26: 93–98.

Bear, M. and Moody, L. (1990) Formulating research questions or hypotheses, chapter 5 in Moody, L.E. (1990) *Advancing Nursing Science through Research*, Volume 1, London: Sage, pp.146–183.

Beaver, K. and Luker, K. (1997) Readability of patient information booklets for women with breast cancer, *Patient Education and Counseling*, 31: 95–102.

Becker, M.H. and Maiman, L.A. (1975) Sociobehavioural determinants of compliance with medical care regimens, *Medical Care*, 13: 10–24.

Becker, M.H. and Rosenstock, I.M. (1984) Compliance with medical advice, chapter 6 in Steptoe, S.A. and Mathews, A. (eds) *Health Care and Human Behaviour*, London: Academic Press, pp. 175–208.

Benner, P. (1984) *From Novice to Expert: Excellence and Power in Clinical Nursing Practice*, Menlo Park: Addison-Wesley Publishing Company.

Benoliel, J.Q. (1984) Advancing nursing science: qualitative approaches, *Western Journal of Nursing Research*, 6(3): 1–8.

Berg, B.L. (1989) *Qualitative Research Methods for the Social Sciences*, Boston: Allyn and Bacon.

Bernier, M.J. (1992) Current perspectives: psychoeducation: subset or prototype of the health education model?, *Patient Education and Counseling*, 19: 125–127.

Bernier, M.J. (1993) Developing and evaluating printed education materials. A prescriptive model for quality, *Orthopaedic Nursing*, 12: 39–45.

Biley, F.C. (1992) Some determinants that effect patient participation in decision making about nursing care, *Journal of Advanced Nursing* 17: 414–421.

Biley, F.C. and Wright, S.G. (1997) Towards a defence of nursing routine and ritual, *Journal of Clinical Nursing*, 6: 115–119.

Binik, Y.M., Devins, G.D., Barre, P.E., Guttman, R.D., Hollomby, D.J., Mandin, H., Leendert, C.P., Hons, R.B. and Burgess, E.D. (1993) Live and learn: patient education delays the need to initiate renal replacement therapy in end-stage renal disease, *Journal of Nervous Mental Disease*, 181(6): 371–376.

Bircumshaw, D. (1990) The utilization of research findings in clinical nursing practice, *Journal of Advanced Nursing*, 15: 1272–1280.

Bird, S.T., Earp, J.A.L., Drezner, S.M. and Cooper, H. (1994) Patient education for sickle cell disease: a national survey of health care professionals, *Health Education Research*, 9(2): 235–242.

Boore, J.R.P. (1978) *Prescription for Recovery*, London: Royal College of Nursing.

Booth, B. (1992) Nursing diagnosis: one step forward, *Nursing Times*, 88(7): 31–32.

Bosley, C.M., Fosbury, J.A. and Cochrane, G.M. (1995) The psychological factors associated with poor compliance with treatment in asthma, *European Respiratory Journal*, 8(6): 899–904.

Bostrom, J., Crawford-Swent, C., Lazar, N. and Helmer, D. (1994) Learning needs of hospitalized and recently discharged patients, *Patient Education and Counseling*, 23: 83–89.

Bradley, C. (ed.) (1994) *Handbook of Psychology and Diabetes*, Switzerland: Harwood Academic Publishers.

Brearley, S. (1990) *Patient participation: the literature*, Middlesex: Scutari Press.

Breemhaar, B., van den Borne, H.W. and Mullen, P.D. (1996) Inadequacies of surgical patient education, *Patient Education and Counseling*, 28: 31–44.

Brody, D.S. (1980) The patient's role in clinical decision-making, *Annals of Internal Medicine* 83: 718–722.

Broome, A. and Llewelyn, S. (eds) (1995) *Health Psychology: Processes and Applications*, Edinburgh: Chapman and Hall.

Brown, S. (1990) Studies of educational interventions and outcomes in diabetic adults: a meta-analysis revisited, *Patient Education and Counseling*, 16: 189–215.

Brown, S.A. (1990) Quality of reporting in diabetes patient education research: 1954–1986, *Research in Nursing and Health*, 13: 53–62.

Brownlea, A. (1987) Participation: myths, realities, and progress, *Social Science and Medicine*, 25(6); 605–614.

Brownlee-Duffeck, M., Peterson, L., Simonds, J.F., Goldstein, D., Kilo, C. and Hoette, S. (1987) The role of health beliefs in the regimen adherence and metabolic control of adolescents and adults with diabetes mellitus, *Journal of Consulting and Clinical Psychology*, 55(2): 139–144.

Bruce, S.L. and Grove, S.K. (1994) The effect of a coronary artery risk evaluation program on serum lipid values and cardiovascular risk levels, *Applied Nursing Research*, 7(2): 67–74.

Bubela, N., Galloway, S., McCay, E., McKibbon, A., Nagle, L., Pringle, D., Ross, E. and Shamain, J. (1990) Factors influencing patients' informational needs at time of hospital discharge, *Patient Education and Counseling*, 16: 21–28.

Buchan, J. (1992) Cost-effective caring, *International Nursing Review*, 39(4): 117–120.

Buchanan, B.G., Moore, J.D., Forsythe, D.E., Carenini, G., Ohlsson, S. and Banks, G. (1995) An intelligent interactive system for delivering individualised information to patients, *Artificial Intelligence in Medicine*, 7: 117–154.

Burckhardt, C.S. [Taskforce chairperson and representative of the Arthritis Foundation] (1994) Arthritis and musculoskeletal patient education standards, Special Report/Editorial, *Arthritis Care and Research*, 7(1): 1–4.

Busby, A. and Gilchrist, B. (1992) The role of the nurse in the medical ward round, *Journal of Advanced Nursing*, 17: 339–346.

Butow, P., Brindle, E., McConnell, D., Boakes, R. and Tattersall, M. (1998) Information booklets about cancer: factors influencing patient satisfaction and utilisation, *Patient Education and Counseling*, 33: 129–141.

Byrne, D.J., Napier, A. and Cuschieri, A. (1988) How informed is signed consent?, *British Medical Journal*, 296: 839–840.

Calnan, M. (1995) The role of the general practitioner in health promotion in the UK: the case of coronary heart disease prevention, *Patient Education and Counseling*, 25: 301–304.

Cameron, C. (1996) Patient compliance: recognition of factors involved and suggestions for promoting compliance with therapeutic regimens, *Journal of Advanced Nursing*, 24: 244–250.

Cameron, K. and Gregor, F. (1987) Chronic illness and compliance, *Journal of Advanced Nursing*, 12: 671–676.

Cameron, R. and Best, A. (1987) Promoting adherence to health behaviour change interventions: recent findings from behavioural research, *Patient Education and Counseling*, 10: 139–154.

Camiah, S. (1997) Utilization of nursing research in practice and application strategies to raise research awareness amongst nurse practitioners: a model for success, *Journal of Advanced Nursing*, 26: 1193–1202.

Caraher, M. (1994) Nursing and health promotion practice: the creation of victims and winners in a political context, *Journal of Advanced Nursing*, 19: 465–468.

Caraher, M. (1998) Patient education and health promotion: clinical health promotion – the conceptual link, *Patient Education and Counseling*, 33: 49–58.

Carmines, E.G. (1986) The analysis of co-variance structure models. Chapter 2 in Berry, W.D. and Lewis Beck, M.S. (eds) *New Tools for Social Scientists. Advances and Applications in Research Methods*, London: Sage.

Carnevali, D.L. and Thomas, M.D. (1993) *Diagnostic Reasoning and Treatment Decision-Making in Nursing*, Philadelphia: J.B. Lippincott Company.

Caron, H.S. (1985) Compliance: the case for objective measurement, *Journal of Hypertension*, 3, Supplement 1: 11–17.

Carper, B.A. (1978) Fundamental patterns of knowing in nursing, *Advances in Nursing Science*, 1: 13–23.

Cartwright, A. (1964) *Human Relations and Hospital Care*, London: Routledge & Kegan Paul.

Castledine, G. (1985) Guidelines for success, *Nursing Times*, 81(21): 22.

Chapman, G., Elstein, A. and Hughes, K. (1995) Effects of patient education on decisions about breast cancer treatments, *Medical Decision Making*, 15(3): 231–239.

Chavasse, J. (1992) New dimensions of empowerment in nursing and challenges, *Journal of Advanced Nursing*, 17(1): 1–2.

Cherkin, D.C., Deyo, R.A., Street, J.H., Hunt, M. and Barlow, W. (1996) Limited success of a program for back pain in primary care, *Spine*, 21(3): 345–355.

Clark, C.J. (1994) The influence of education on morbidity and mortality in asthma (including the use of open access hospital admission for severe attacks), *Monaldi Archives for Chest Disease*, 49(2): 169–172.

Clark, J. (1997) Virginia Henderson Memorial Lecture: Keynote Address, International Congress of Nurses, ICN 21st Quadrennial Congress, Vancouver 15–20 June.

Clarke, L. (1992) Qualitative research: meaning and language, *Journal of Advanced Nursing*, 17: 243–252.

Clay, T. (1987) *Nurses: Power and Politics*, London: Heinemann Nursing.

Clement, S. (1995) Diabetes self-management education, *Diabetes Care*, 18(8): 1204–1214.

Clifford, C. (1993) The role of nurse teachers in the empowerment of nurses through research, *Nurse Education Today*, 13: 47–54.

Close, A. (1988) Patient education: a literature review, *Journal of Advanced Nursing*, 13: 203–213.

Coates, V.E. (1993) *Beliefs, Knowledge and the Self-management of Diabetes*, Doctor of Philosophy Thesis, University of Ulster.

Coates, V.E. and Boore, J.R.P. (1995) Self-management of chronic illness: implications for nursing, *International Journal of Nursing Studies*, 32(6): 628–640.

Coates, V.E. and Boore, J.R.P. (1996) Knowledge and diabetes self-management, *Patient Education and Counseling*, 29: 99–108.

Coey, L. (1996) Readability of printed educational materials used to perform potential and actual ostomates, *Journal of Clinical Nursing*, 5(6): 359–366.

Cohen, L. and Manion, L. (1980) *Research Methods in Education*, London: Croom Helm.

Coles, C.R. (1989) Diabetes education: theories of practice, *Practical Diabetes*, 6: 199–202.

Conner, M. and Norman, P. (1996) *Predicting Health Behaviour*, Buckingham: Open University Press.

Coonrod, B.A., Harris, M.I. and Betschart, J. (1994) Frequency and determinants of diabetes patient education among adults in the U.S. population, *Diabetes Care*, 17(8): 852–858.

Cormack, D.F.S. (ed.) (1996) *The Research Process in Nursing*, Oxford: Blackwell Science.

Cramer, J.A. (1991) Overview of methods to measure and enhance patient compliance, chapter 1 in Cramer, J.A. and Spilker, B. (eds) (1991) *Patient Compliance in Medical Practice and Clinical Trials*, New York: Raven Press.

Cramer, J.A. and Spilker, B. (eds) (1991) *Patient Compliance in Medical Practice and Clinical Trials*, New York: Raven Press.

Crate, M.A. (1965) Nursing functions in adaptation to chronic illness, *American Journal of Nursing*, 65: 72–76.

Dalayon, A.P. (1994) Components of preoperative patient teaching in Kuwait, *Journal of Advanced Nursing*, 19: 537–542.

Davis, M.S. (1968) Variations in patient's compliance with doctor's advice: an empirical analysis of patterns of communication, *American Journal of Public Health*, 58(2): 274–288.

Davis, T.C., Jackson, R.H., George, R.B., Long, S.W., Talley, D., Murphy, P.W., Mayeaux, E.J. and Truong, T. (1993) Reading ability in patients in substance misuse treatment centers, *The International Journal of the Addictions*, 28(6): 571–582.

Davis, T.C., Mayeaux, E.J., Frederickson, D., Bocchini, J.A., Jackson, R.H. and Murphy, P.W. (1994) Reading ability of parents compared with reading level of pediatrics patient education materials, *Pediatrics*, 93(3): 460–468.

De Muth, J.S. (1989) Patient teaching in the ambulatory setting, *Nursing Clinics of North America*, 24(3): 645–654.

Deane, D.M. (1991) Content, construct, and criterion-related validity, *The Diabetes Educator*, 17(5): 361–362.

Dearoff, W.W. (1986) Computerized health education: a comparison with traditional formats, *Health Education Quarterly*, 13: 61–72.

Department of Health (1992a) *The Health of the Nation*, London: HMSO.

Department of Health (1992b) *The Patients' Charter*, London: HMSO.

Department of Health (1993) *A Vision for the Future*, London: HMSO.

Department of Health (1994) *The Challenges for Nursing and Midwifery in the 21st Century – The Heathrow Report*, London: HMSO.

Department of Health (1995) *On the State of the Public Health. The Annual Report of the Chief Medical Officer of the Department of Health for the Year 1994*, London: HMSO.

Department of Health (1997) *The New NHS: Modern – Dependable*, Cm3807, London: HMSO.

Department of Health (Secretaries of State for Health, Wales, Northern Ireland, and Scotland) (1989) *Working for Patients*, London: HMSO.

Derdiarian, A.K. (1986) Informational needs of recently diagnosed cancer patients, *Nursing Research*, 35(5): 276–281.

DeVellis, R.F. and Blalock, S.J. (1993) Psychological and educational interventions to reduce arthritis disability, *Bailliere's Clinical Rheumatology*, 7(2): 397–416.

Devine, E.C. and Westlake, S.K. (1995) The effects of psychoeducational care provided to adults with cancer: meta-analysis of 116 studies, *Oncology Nursing Forum*, 22(9): 1369–1381.

Dickson, D., Hargie, O. and Morrow, N. (1997) *Communication Skills Training for Health Professionals*, 2nd edition, London: Chapman & Hall.

Didlake, R.H., Dreyfus, K., Kerman, R.H., Van Burenc, T. and Kahan, B.D. (1988) Patient non-compliance: a major cause of late graft failure in cyclosporin-treated renal transplants, *Transplantation Proceedings*, 20: 63–69.

DiMatteo, M.R. and DiNicola, D.D. (1982) *Achieving Patient Compliance: The Psychology of the Medical Practitioner's Role*, New York, Oxford: Pergamon Press.

Dollahite, J., Thompson, C. and McNew, R. (1996) Readability of printed sources of diet and health information, *Patient Education and Counseling*, 27: 123–134.

D'Onofrio, C.N. (1980) Patient compliance and patient education: some fundamental issues, chapter 15 in Squyres, W.D. (ed.) *Patient Education: An Inquiry into the State of the Art*, New York: Springer Publishing Company.

Draper, P. (1996) Compromise, massive encouragement and forcing: a discussion of mechanisms used to limit the choices available to the older adult in hospital, *Journal of Clinical Nursing*, 5: 325–331.

Droogan, J. and Song, F. (1996) The process and importance of systematic reviews, *Nurse Researcher*, 4(1): 15–26.

Dubach, E. and Nendick, P. (1986) No frills patient education, *Canadian Nurse*, 82: 21–23.

Duffy, M.E. (1985) A research appraisal checklist for evaluating nursing research reports, *Nursing and Health Care*, 6: 539–547.

Dunn, S. (1988) Treatment-education, *Bailliere's Clinical Endocrinology and Metabolism*, 2: 493–506.

Dunn, S.M. (1995) Barriers and challenges in training health care providers for patient education, *Patient Education and Counseling*, 26: 131–138.

Dunn, S.M., Beeney, L.J., Hoskins, P.L. and Turtle, J.R. (1990) Knowledge and attitude change as predictors of metabolic improvement in diabetes education, *Social Science and Medicine*, 31: 1135–1141.

Dunn, S.M., Bryson, J.M., Hoskin, P.L., Alford, J.B., Handelsman, D.J. and Turtle, J.R. (1984) Development of the diabetes knowledge (DKN) scales: forms DKNa, DKNb, DKNc, *Diabetes Care*, 7: 36–41.

Dunn, V., Crichton, N., Roe, B., Seers, K. and Williams, K. (1998) Using research for practice: a UK experience of the BARRIERS Scale, *Journal of Advanced Nursing*, 27: 1203–1210.

Dzurec, L.C. (1990) Research to understand living with diabetes, *The Diabetes Educator*, 16(4): 276–281.

Edwards, M.H. (1990) Satisfying patients' needs for surgical information, *British Journal of Surgery*, 77: 463–465.

Engel, G.L. (1977) The need for a new medical model. A challenge for biomedicine, *Science*, 196(4286): 129–136.

Engle, G.L. (1964) Grief and grieving, *American Journal of Nursing*, 64: 93–98.

Engstrom, F.W. (1991) Clinical correlates of antidepressant compliance, chapter 15 in Cramer, J.A. and Spilker, B. (eds) (1991) *Patient Compliance in Medical Practice and Clinical Trials*, New York: Raven Press, pp. 187–194.

Fahrenfort, M. (1987) Patient emancipation by health education: an impossible goal?, *Patient Education and Counseling*, 10: 25–37.

Fain, J.A. (1995) Editorial: Making things happen, *The Diabetes Educator*, 21(6): 503.

Falvo, D.R. (1985) *Effective Patient Education: A Guide to Increased Compliance*, Maryland: Aspen Publications.

Falvo, D.R. (1995) Educational evaluation: what are the outcomes?, *Advances in Renal Replacement Therapy*, 2(3): 227–233.

Faulkner, A. (1993) *Teaching Effective Interaction in Health Care*, London: Chapman Hall.

Faulkner, A. (1994) Using simulators to aid the teaching of communication skills in cancer and palliative care, *Patient Education and Counseling*, 23: 125–129.

Faulkner, A., Webb, P. and Maguire, P. (1991) Communication and counseling skills: educating health professionals working in cancer palliative care. *Patient Education and Counseling*, 18: 3–7.

Fawcett, J. (1992) Contemporary conceptualizations of nursing: philosophy or science?, chapter 6 in Kikuchi, J.F. and Simmons, H. (eds) *Philosophic Inquiry in Nursing*, London: Sage.

Fawzy, F.I. (1995) A short-term psychoeducational intervention for patients newly diagnosed with cancer, *Support Care Cancer* (Germany), 3: 235–238.

Ferrell, B.R., Ferrell, B.A., Ahn, C. and Tran, K. (1994) Pain management for elderly patients with cancer at home, *Cancer: Supplement*, 74(7): 2139–2146.

Feste, C. and Anderson, R.M. (1995) Empowerment: from philosophy to practice, *Patient Education and Counseling*, 26: 139–144.

Fishbein, M. and Ajzen, I. (1975) *Belief, Attitude, Intention and Behaviour*, Reading, Mass: Addison-Wesley.

Fisher, R.C. (1992) Patient education and compliance: a pharmacist's perspective, *Patient Education and Counseling*, 19: 261–271.

Fitzgerald, T.M. and Glotzer, D.E. (1995) Vaccine information pamphlets: more information than parents want?, *Pediatrics US*, 95(3): 331–334.

Fitzpatrick, R., Hinton, J., Newman, S., Scambler, G. and Thompson, J. (1984) *The Experience of Illness*, Tavistock Publications: London.

Flaherty, M. (1981) For Mara, *Nursing Mirror*, 152(9): 24–26.

Flesch, R. (1974) *The Art of Readable Writing*, New York: Harper & Row, pp. 184–186, 247–251.

Folkman, S. and Lazarus, R.S. (1985) If it changes it must be a process: a study of emotion and coping during three stages of a college examination, *Journal of Personality and Social Psychiatry*, 48: 150–170.

Ford, P. and Walsh, M. (1994) *New Rituals for Old: Nursing through the Looking Glass*, Oxford: Butterworth-Heinemann.

Frederikson, L.G. (1993) Development of an integrative model for medical consultation, *Health Communication*, 5: 225–237.

Frederikson, L.G. (1995) Exploring information-exchange in consultation: the patients' view of performance and outcomes, *Patient Education and Counseling*, 25: 237–246.

Frederikson, L.G. and Bull, P.E. (1995) Evaluation of a patient education leaflet designed to improve communication in medical consultations, *Patient Education and Counseling*, 25: 51–57.

Fredette, S.L. (1990) A model for improving cancer patient education, *Cancer Nursing*, 13(4): 207–215.

French, B. (1997) British studies which measure patient outcome, 1990–1994, *Journal of Advanced Nursing*, 26: 320–328.

Fries, J.F., Carey, C. and McChane, D.J. (1997) Patient education in arthritis: randomized controlled trial of a mail-delivered program, *The Journal of Rheumatology*, 24(7): 1378–1383.

Funk, S.G., Champagne, M.T., Wiese, R.A. and Tornquist, E.M. (1991) BARRIERS: The barriers to research utilization scale, *Applied Nursing Research*, 4(2): 90–95.

Funnell, M., Anderson, R., Arnold, M., Barr, P., Donnelly, M., Johnson, P., Taylor-Moon, D. and White, N.H. (1990) Empowerment: an idea whose time has come in diabetes education, *The Diabetes Educator*, 17(1): 37–41.

Gagne, R.M. (1965) *The Conditions of Learning*, New York: Holt, Rinehart and Winston.

Gagne, R.M. (1972) Domains of learning, *Interchange*, III: 1–8.

Ganong, L.A. (1987) Integrative reviews of nursing research, *Research in Nursing and Health*, 10: 1–11.

Gibbs, S., Waters, W.E. and George, C.F. (1989) The benefits of prescription information leaflets, *British Journal of Clinical Pharmacology*, 27: 723–739.

Glasgow, R., La Chance, P., Toobert, D., Brown, J., Hampson, S. and Riddle, M. (1997) Long term effects and costs of brief behavioural dietary intervention for patients with diabetes delivered from the medical office, *Patient Education and Counseling*, 32: 175–184.

Glasgow, R.E. and Osteen, V.L. (1992) Evaluating diabetes education. Are we measuring the most important outcomes?, *Diabetes Care*, 15(10): 1423–1432.

Glimelius, B., Birgegard, G., Hoffman, K., Kvale, G. and Sjoden, P. (1995) Information to and communication with cancer patients: improvements and psychosocial correlates in a comprehensive care program for patients and their relatives, *Patient Education and Counseling*, 25: 171–182.

Goodall, T. and Halford, W. (1991) Self-management of diabetes mellitus: a critical review, *Health Psychology*, 10(1): 1–8.

Goode, C.J., Lovett, M.K., Hayes, J.E. and Butcher, L.A. (1987) Use of research based knowledge in clinical practice, *Journal of Nursing Administration*, 17(12): 11–18.

Goodman, H. (1997) Patients' perceptions of their education needs in the first six weeks following discharge after cardiac surgery, *Journal of Advanced Nursing*, 25: 1241–1251.

Goodwin, L.D. and Goodwin, W.L. (1991) Focus on psychometrics: estimating construct validity, *Research in Nursing and Health*, 14: 235–243.

Gordis, L. (1976) Methodological issues in the measurement of patient compliance, chapter 5 in Sackett, D.L. and Haynes, R.B. (eds)

Compliance with Therapeutic Regimens, Baltimore and London: The Johns Hopkins University Press.

Gordon, M. (1994) *Nursing Diagnosis: Process and Application*, 3rd edition, St. Louis: Mosby.

Graveley, E.A. and Oseasohn, C.S. (1991) Multiple drug regimens: medication compliance among veterans 65 years and over, *Research in Nursing and Health*, 14: 51–58.

Gray, G. and Pratt, G. (1991) Prologue in Gray, G. and Pratt, R. (eds) *Towards a Discipline of Nursing*, Edinburgh: Churchill Livingstone, pp. 1–9.

Graydon, J., Galloway, S., Palmer-Wickham, S., Harrison, D., Rich-van der Bij, L., West, P., Burlein-Hall, S. and Evans-Boyden, B. (1997) Information needs of women during early treatment for breast cancer, *Journal of Advanced Nursing*, 26: 59–64.

Green, L.W., Kreuter, M.W., Partridge, K.B. and Deeds, S.G. (1979) *Health Education Planning: A Diagnostic Approach*, Palo Alto: Mayfield.

Greenfield, S., Kaplan, S. and Ware, J.E. (1985) Expanding patient involvement in care, *Annals of Internal Medicine*, 102: 520–528.

Griffiths, P. (1995) Progress in measuring nursing outcomes, *Journal of Advanced Nursing*, 21: 1092–1100.

Gruninger, U. (1995) Patient education: an example of one-to-one communication, *Journal of Human Hypertension*, 9: 15–25.

Gunning, R. (1968) *The Technique of Clear Writing*, New York: McGraw-Hill.

Hack, T.F., Degner, L.F. and Dyck, D.G. (1994) Relationship between preferences for decisional control and illness information among women with breast cancer: a quantitive and qualitative analysis, *Social Science and Medicine*, 39(2): 279–289.

Hagenhoff, B.D., Feutz, C., Conn, V.S., Sagehorn, K.K. and Moranville-Hunziker, M. (1994) Patient education needs as reported by congestive heart failure patients and their nurses, *Journal of Advanced Nursing*, 19: 685–690.

Hathaway, D. (1986) Effect of preoperative instruction on postoperative outcomes: a meta-analysis, *Nursing Research*, 35(5): 269–275.

Hawley, D.J. (1995) Psycho-educational interventions in the treatment of arthritis, *Bailliere's Clinical Rheumatology*, 9(4): 803–823.

Haynes, R.B., Wang, E. and Gomes, M. (1987) A critical review of interventions to improve compliance with prescribed medications, *Patient Education and Counseling*, 10: 155–166.

Hayward, J. (1975) *Information – A Prescription Against Pain*, London: Royal College of Nursing.

Hearth-Holmes, M., Murphy, P., Davis, T., Nandy, I., Elder, C., Broadwell, L. and Wolf, R. (1997) Literacy in patients with a chronic disease: systemic lupus erythematosus and the reading level of patient education materials, *The Journal of Rheumatology*, 24(12): 2335–2339.

Henderson, V. (1966) *The Nature of Nursing. A Definition and its Implications for Practice, Research, and Education*, New York: Macmillan.

Hendricks, J. and Baume, P. (1997) The pricing of nursing care, *Journal of Advanced Nursing*, 27: 454–462.

Herbert, C.P. (1996) Patient information for improved self care: a critical appraisal, *Patient Education and Counseling*, 27: 121–122.

Herbert, C.P. (1997) The relevance of cultural diversity to patient education, *Patient Education and Counseling*, 31: Editorial.

Hewison, A. (1995) Nurses' power in interactions with patients, *Journal of Advanced Nursing*, 21: 75–82.

Hicks, C. and Hennessy, D. (1997) Mixed messages in nursing research: their contribution to the persisting hiatus between evidence and practice, *Journal of Advanced Nursing*, 25: 595–601.

Higgins, L. and Ambrose, P. (1995) The effect of adjunct questions on older adults' recall of information from a patient education booklet, *Patient Education and Counseling*, 25: 67–74.

Hill, J. (1997) A practical guide to patient education and information giving, *Bailliere's Clinical Rheumatology*, 11(1): 109–127.

Hilton, S., Sibbald, B., Anderson, H.R. and Freeling, P. (1986) Controlled evaluation of the effects of patient education on asthma morbidity in general practice, *Lancet*, 1(8471): 26–29.

Hirano, P.C., Laurent, D.D. and Lorig, K. (1994) Arthritis patient education studies 1987–1991: a review of the literature, *Patient Education and Counseling*, 24: 9–54.

HMSO (1972) Report of the Committee on Nursing (Briggs Report) Cmnd 5115, London: HMSO.

Hogston, R. (1997) Nursing diagnosis and classification systems: a position paper, *Journal of Advanced Nursing*, 26: 496–500.

Holmes, C. (1991) Theory: where are we going and what have we missed along the way?, Chapter 21 in Gray, G. and Pratt, R. (eds) *Towards a Discipline of Nursing*, Edinburgh: Churchill Livingstone, pp. 435–460.

Honan, S., Krsnak, G., Petersen, D. and Torkelson, R. (1988) The nurse as patient educator: perceived responsibilities and factors enhancing role development, *The Journal of Continuing Education in Nursing*, 19(1): 33–37.

Honey, P. and Mumford, A. (1986) *Using your Learning Styles*, 2nd edition, Maidenhead: Peter Honey.

Hulka, B.S., Kupper, L.L., Cassel, J.C. and Babineau, R.A. (1975b) Practice characteristics and quality of primary medical care, *Medical Care*, 13: 808–820.

Hulka, B.S., Kupper, L.L., Cassel, J.C. and Mayo, F. (1975a) Doctor-patient communication and outcomes among diabetic patients, *Journal of Community Health*, 1: 15–27.

Hunt, M. (1987) The process of translating research findings into nursing practice, *Journal of Advanced Nursing*, 12: 101–110.

Hunter, D. (1996) Effective Practice. Refocus the NHS Executive, *Northern and Yorkshire Research and Development Newsletter*, Issue 2, Summer: 4–5.

Jaarsma, T., Kastermans, M., Dassen, T. and Philipsen, H. (1995) Problems of cardiac patients in early recovery, *Journal of Advanced Nursing*, 21: 21–27.

Jackson, R.H., Davis, T.C., Murphy, P., Bairnsfather, L.E. and George, R.B. (1994) Reading deficiencies in older patients, *The American Journal of the Medical Sciences*, 308(2): 79–82.

Janz, N.K. and Becker, M.H. (1984) The Health Belief Model: a decade later, *Health Education Quarterly*, 11(1): 1–47.

Jarvis, P. and Gibson, S. (1985) *The Teacher Practitioner in Nursing, Midwifery and Health Visiting*, London: Croom Helm.

Jenkins, C.D. (1995) An integrated behavioural medicine approach to improving care of patients with diabetes mellitus, *Behavioural Medicine*, 21(2): 53–65.

Jenny, J. (1978) A strategy for patient teaching, *Journal of Advanced Nursing*, 3: 341–348.

Jenny, J. (1990) Nursing patient education: a Canadian perspective, *Patient Education and Counseling*, 16: 47–52.

Jimison, H., Fagan, L., Shachter, R. and Shortliffe, E. (1992) Patient-specific explanation in models of chronic disease, *Artificial Intelligence in Medicine*, 4: 191–205.

Jones, S.L., Jones, P.K. and Katz, J. (1991) Compliance in acute and chronic patients receiving a Health Belief Model intervention in the emergency department, *Social Science and Medicine*, 32(10): 1183–1189.

Kahn, G. (1993) Computer-based patient education: a progress report, *M.D. Computing*, 10(2): 93–99.

Kappeli, S. (1993) Advanced clinical practice – how do we promote it?, *Journal of Clinical Nursing*, 2: 205–210.

Kemp, N. and Richardson, E. (1994) *The Nursing Process and Quality Care*, London: Edward Arnold.

Kiger, A.M. (1995) *Teaching for Health*, 2nd edition, Edinburgh: Churchill Livingstone.

King's Fund (1996) *The Cost of Non-insulin Diabetes Mellitus*, London: British Diabetic Association.

Knafl, K.A. and Breitmayer, B.J. (1991) Triangulation in qualitative research: issues of conceptual clarity and purpose, Chapter 13 in Morse, J.M. (ed.) *Qualitative Nursing Research*, London: Sage.

Knowles, M.S. (1980) The modern practice of adult education: from pedagogy to andragogy, 2nd edition, Chicago: Follett.

Knowles, M.S. (1990) *The Adult Learner: A Neglected Species*, 4th edition, Houston: Gulf Publishing.

Kolb, D.A. (1976) *Learning Styles Inventory: Technical Manual*, Boston: McBer & Co.

Krantz, D.S., Baum, A. and Wideman, M. (1980) Assessment of preferences for self-treatment and information in health care, *Journal of Personality and Social Psychology*, 39(5): 977–990.

Krishna, S., Balas, A., Spencer, D., Griffin, J. and Austin Boren, S. (1997) Clinical trials of interactive computerized patient education: implications for family practice, *The Journal of Family Practice*, 45(1): 25–33.

Kubler-Ross, E. (1969) *On Death and Dying*, New York: Macmillan.

Kyngas, H. and Hentinen, M. (1995) Meaning attached to compliance with self-care, and conditions for compliance among young diabetics, *Journal of Advanced Nursing*, 21: 729–736.

Lacey, A.E. (1994) Research utilization in nursing practice – a pilot study, *Journal of Advanced Nursing*, 19: 987–995.

Latter, S., Macleod Clark, J., Wilson-Barnett, J. and Maben, J. (1992) Health education in nursing: perceptions of practice in acute settings, *Journal of Advanced Nursing*, 17: 164–172.

Lauer, P., Murphy, S.P. and Powers, M.J. (1982) Learning needs of cancer patients: a comparison of nurse and patient perceptions, *Nursing Research*, 31(1): 11–16.

Le May, M. (1998) *Empowering Older People through Communication*, chapter 4 in Kendall, S. (ed.) *Health and Empowerment*, London: Arnold, pp. 91–111.

LeCompte, M.D. and Goetz, J.P. (1982) Problems of reliability and validity in ethnographic research, *Review of Ethnographic Research*, 52(1): 31–60.

Leininger, M.M. (1987) Importance and uses of ethnomethods: ethnography and ethnonursing research, in Cahoon, M.C. (ed.) *Recent Advances in Nursing 17*, Edinburgh: Churchill Livingstone.

Leirer, V.O., Morrow, D.G., Pariante, G.M. and Sheikh, J.I. (1988) Elders' nonadherence, its assessment, and computer assisted instruction for medication recall training, *Journal American Geriatric Society*, 36: 877–884.

Leventhal, H. and Cameron, L. (1987) Behavioural theories and the problem of compliance, *Patient Education and Counseling*, 10: 117–138.

Leventhal, H., Nerenz, D.R. and Steele, D.J. (1984) Illness representations and coping with health threats, in Baum, A. and Singer, J. (ed.) *A Handbook of Psychology and Health*, Hillsdale, NJ: Erlbaum Associates, pp. 219–252.

Lewis, D. (1996) Computer-based patient education: use by diabetes educators, *The Diabetes Educator*, 22(2): 140–145.

Ley, P. (1982) Giving information to patients, chapter 14 in Eiser, J.R. (ed.) *Social Psychology and Behavioural Medicine*, Chichester: John Wiley and Sons, pp. 339–373.

Ley, P. (1988) *Communicating with Patients*, London: Chapman and Hall.

Liljas, B. and Lahdensuo, A. (1997) Is asthma self-management cost-effective?, *Patient Education and Counseling*, 32: S97–S104.

Lindeman, C.A. (1988) Patient education, *Annual Review of Nursing Research*, 6: 29–60.

Lisper, L., Isacson, D., Sjoden, P. and Bingefors, K. (1997) Medicated hypertensive patients' views and experience of information and communication concerning antihypertensive drugs, *Patient Education and Counseling*, 32: 147–155.

Little, D.E. and Carnevali, D.L. (1976) *Nursing Care Planning*, 2nd edition, Philadelphia: J.B. Lippincott.

Lorig, K. (1995) Patient education: treatment or nice extra, *British Society for Rheumatology*, 34: 703–706.

Lorig, K. and Visser, A. (1994) Editorial: Arthritis patient education standards: a model for the future, *Patient Education and Counseling*, 24: 3–7.

Lovell, R.B. (1980) *Adult Learning*, London: Croom Helm.

Luker, K. and Kendrick, M. (1995) Towards knowledge-based practice: an evaluation of a method of dissemination, *International Journal of Nursing Studies*, 32(1): 59–67.

Luker, K.A. and Caress, A. (1989) Rethinking patient education, *Journal of Advanced Nursing*, 14: 711–718.

Luker, K.A. and Caress, A. (1991) The development and evaluation of computer assisted learning for patients on continuous ambulatory peritoneal dialysis, *Computers in Nursing*, 9(1): 15–21.

Lutzen, K. and Tishelman, C. (1996) Nursing diagnosis: a critical analysis of underlying assumptions, *International Journal of Nursing*, 33(2): 190–200.

Maguire, P., Roe, P., Goldberg, D., Jones, S., Hyde, C. and O'Dowd, T. (1978) The value of feedback in teaching interviewing skills to medical students, *Psychological Medicine*, 8: 695–704.

Mahoney, C.D. *et al.* (1983) Recorded medication messages for ambulatory patients, *American Journal of Hospital Pharmacy*, 40: 448–449.

Marks, I.M., Hallam, R.S., Connolly, J. and Philpott, R. (1977) *Nursing in Behavioural Psychotherapy*, RCN: London.

Marks-Maran, D.J., Docking, S.P., Maunder, T. and Scott, J. (1988) *Skills for Care Planning*, London: Scutari Press.

Maslow, A. (1970) *Motivation and Personality*, London: Harper and Row.

May, C. (1995) Patient autonomy and the politics of professional relationships, *Journal of Advanced Nursing*, 21: 83–87.

Mayeaux, E., Murphy, P., Arnold, C., Davis, T., Jackson, R.H. and Sentell, T. (1996) Improving patient education for patients with low literacy skills, *American Family Physician*, 53(1): 205–211.

McFarland, G.K. and McFarlane, E.A. (1989) *Nursing Diagnosis and Intervention: Planning for Patient Care*, St. Louis: Mosby.

McKenna, H.P. (1995) Nursing skill mix substitutions and quality of care: an exploration of assumptions from the research literature, *Journal of Advanced Nursing*, 21: 452–459.

McLaughlin, G. (1969) SMOG grading – a new readability formula, *Journal of Reading*, 12: 639–646.

Meeker, B.J. (1994) Preoperative patient education: evaluating post-operative patient outcomes, *Patient Education and Counseling*, 23: 41–47.

Meerabeau, L. (1992) Tacit nursing knowledge: an untapped resource or a methodological headache?, *Journal of Advanced Nursing*, 17: 108–112.

Meissner, H.I., Anderson, M. and Odenkirchen, J.C. (1990) Meeting information needs of significant others: use of the Cancer Information Service, *Patient Education and Counseling*, 15: 171–179.

Menzies, I. (1960) A case study in the functioning of social systems as a defence against anxiety, *Human Relations*, 13: 95–121.

Merriam, S.B. (1987) Adult learning and theory building: a review, *Adult Education Quarterly*, 37(4): 187–198.

Merriam, S.B. (1988) Finding your way through the maze, *Lifelong Learning: an omnibus of practice and research*, 11(6): 4–7.

Messenger, K. (1992) *Clients as Individuals*, Edinburgh: Churchill Livingstone.

Mikulaninec, C.E. (1987) Effects of mailed preoperative instructions on learning and anxiety, *Patient Education and Counseling*, 10: 253–265.

Mirolo, B.R., Bunce, I.H., Chapman, M., Olsen, T., Eliadis, P., Hennessy, J.M., Ward, L.C. and Jones, L.C. (1995) Psychosocial benefits of post-mastectomy lymphedema therapy, *Cancer Nursing*, 18(3): 197–205.

Mistiaen, P., Duijnhouwer, E., Wijkel, D., deBont, M. and Veeger, A. (1997) The problems of elderly people at home one week after discharge from an acute care setting, *Journal of Advanced Nursing*, 25: 1233–1240.

Montgomery, E.B., Lieberman, A., Singh, G., Fries, J.F. and the remaining members of the PROPATH Advisory Board (1994) Patient education and health promotion can be effective in Parkinson's Disease: a randomized controlled trial, *American Journal of Medicine*, 97: 429–435.

Moody, L.E. (1990) *Advancing Nursing Science through Research*, Volume 1, London: Sage.

Moores, Y. (1997) Clinical effectiveness: guest editorial, *Clinical Effectiveness in Nursing*, 1: 3.

Morris, D.B. (1998) Developing a patient education programme: overcoming physician resistance, *The Diabetes Educator*, 24(1): 41–47.

Morse, J.M. and Field, P.A. (1996) *Nursing Research. The Application of Qualitative Approaches*, London: Croom Helm.

Moser, D.K., Dracup, K.A. and Marsden, C. (1993) Needs of recovering cardiac patients and their spouses: compared views, *International Journal of Nursing Studies*, 30(2): 105–114.

Mullen, P.D., Mains, D.A. and Ramon Velez, M.P.H. (1992) A Meta-analysis of controlled trials of cardiac patient education, *Patient Education and Counseling*, 19: 143–162.

Mullen, P.D., Mains, D.A. and Velez, R. (1992) A meta-analysis of controlled trial of cardiac patient education, *Patient Education and Counseling*, 19: 143–162.

Mumford, M. (1997) A descriptive study of the readability of patient information leaflets designed by nurses, *Journal of Advanced Nursing*, 26: 985–991.

Murphy, P.W., Davis, T.C., Jackson, R.H., Decker, B.C. and Long, S.W. (1993) Effects of literacy on health care of the aged: implications for health professionals, *Educational Gerontology*, 19: 311–316.

Naidoo, J. and Wills, J. (1994) *Health Promotion: Foundations for Practice*, London: Bailliere Tindall.

Nathan, R.G., Bont, G.M. and Minz, R.B. (1994) Patient interest in receiving audiotapes of information presented by their physicians, *Archives of Family Medicine*, 3(6): 509–513.

Neufeld, K.R., Degner, L.F. and Dick, J.A.M. (1993) A nursing intervention strategy to foster patient involvement in treatment decisions, *Oncology Nursing Forum*, 20(4): 631–635.

Newell, R. (1994) *Interviewing Skills for Nurses and Other Health Care Professionals*, London: Routledge.

Newell, R. (1996) The reliability and validity of samples, *Nurse Researcher*, 3(4): 16–26.

Nunnally, J.C. (1981) *Psychometric Theory*, New York: McGraw Hill.

Nyhlin, K.T. (1990) A contribution of qualitative research to a better understanding of diabetic patients, *Journal of Advanced Nursing*, 15: 796–803.

O'Brien, B. (1990) Nursing: craft, science and art, in *Conference Proceedings: Dreams, Deliberations and Discoveries: Nursing Research in Action*, Royal Adelaide Hospital, Adelaide, pp. 306–312.

O'Connor, F.W., Devine, E.C., Cook, T.D., Wenk, V.A. and Curtin, T.R. (1990) Enhancing surgical nurses' patient education: development and evaluation of an intervention, *Patient Education and Counseling*, 16: 7–20.

O'Donnell, L.N., Doval, A.S., Duran, R. and O'Donnell, C. (1995) Video-based sexually transmitted disease patient education: its impact on condom acquisition, *American Journal of Public Health*, 85(6): 817–822.

O'Halloran, C.M. and Altmaier, E.M. (1995) The efficacy of preparation for surgery and invasive medical procedures, *Patient Education and Counseling*, 25: 9–16.

Ogier, M.E. (1989) *Working and Learning*, London: Scutari Press.

Ojanlatva, A., Vandenbussche, H.H., Horte, A., Haggblom, T., Kero, J., Kahkonen, J., Mottonen, M., Saraste, A. and Turunen, T. (1997) The use of problem-based learning in dealing with cultural minority groups, *Patient Education and Counseling*, 31: 171–176.

Oldham, J. (1996) Editorial, *Nurse Researcher*, 3(4): 3–4.

Orem, D.E. (1985) *Nursing: Concepts of Practice*, 3rd edition, New York: McGraw Hill.

Osman, L.M., Abdalla, M.I., Beattie, J.A.G., Ross, S.J., Russell, I.T., Friend, J.A., Legge, J.S. and Douglas, J.G. (1994) Reducing hospital admission through computer supported education for asthma patients, *British Medical Journal*, 308: 568–571.

Owens, N.J., Larrant, E.P. amd Fretwell, M.D. (1991) Improving compliance in the older patient: the role of comprehensive functional assessment, chapter 9 in Cramer, J.A. and Spilker, B. (eds) (1991) *Patient Compliance in Medical Practice and Clinical Trials*, New York: Raven Press, pp. 107–119.

Parahoo, K. (1997) *Nursing Research: Principles, Process and Issues*, London: Macmillan Press.

Pender, N.J. (1996) *Health Promotion in Nursing Practice*, 3rd edition, Stamford, Connecticut: Appleton and Lange.

Peplau, H.E. (1952) *Interpersonal Relations in Nursing*, New York: G.P. Putman's Sons.

Peyrot, M., McMurry, J.F. and Hedges, R. (1987) Living with diabetes: the role of personal and professional knowledge in symptom and regimen management. In Roth, J.A. and Conrad, P. (eds) *Research in the Sociology of Health Care. The Experience and Management of Chronic Illness*, JAI Press Inc.: London.

Pohl, M.L. (1965) Teaching activities of the nurse practitioner, *Nursing Research*, 14(1): 4–11.

Polit, D.F. and Hungler, B.P. (1995) *Nursing Research: Principles and Methods* (5th edition), Philadelphia: J.B. Lippincott Company.

Poroch, D. (1995) The effect of preparatory patient education on the anxiety and satisfaction of cancer patients receiving radiation therapy, *Cancer Nursing*, 18(3): 206–214.

Porter, S. (1994) New nursing; the road to freedom, *Journal of Advanced Nursing*, 20: 269–274.

Powell, K.M. and Edgren, B. (1995) Failure of educational videotapes to improve medication compliance in a health maintenance organization, *American Journal of Health System Pharmacy*, 52(20): 2196–2199.

Powers, B.A. and Knapp, T.R. (1990) *A Dictionary of Nursing Theory and Research*, London: Sage Publications.

Pratt, D.D. (1988) Andragogy as a relational concept, *Adult Educational Quarterly*, 38(3): 160–181.

Price, B. (1985) The confidence to educate?, *Nursing Mirror*, 161(17): 39–42.

Prochaska, J.O. and DiClemente, C. (1984) *The Transtheoretical Approach: Crossing Traditional Foundations of Change*, Harnewood, IL: Don Jones/Irwin.

Prochaska, J.O., DiClemente, C. and Norcross, J.C. (1992) In search of how people change: applications to addictive behaviours, *American Psychologist*, 47: 1102–1114.

Radecki, S.E. *et al.* (1989) Telephone patient management by primary care physicians, *Medical Care*, 27: 817–822.

Rankin, S.H. and Stallings, D. (1990) *Patient Education. Issues, Principles, Practices*, Philadelphia: J.B. Lippincott Company.

Raphael, W. (1969) *Patients and their Hospitals*, London: King Edward's Hospital Fund for London.

Rapoff, M.A. and Barnard, M.U. (1991) Compliance with paediatric medical regimens, chapter 7 in Cramer, J.A. and Spilker, B. (eds) (1991) *Patient Compliance in Medical Practice and Clinical Trials*, New York: Raven Press, pp. 73–98.

Redman, B.K. (1984) *The Process of Patient Education*, 5th edition, St. Louis: C.V. Mosby Company.

Redman, B.K. (1988) *The Process of Patient Education*, 6th edition, St. Louis: C.V. Mosby Company.

Redman, B.K. (1993) Patient education at 25 years: where have we been and where are we going?, *Journal of Advanced Nursing*, 18: 725–730.

Reed-Pierce, R. and Cardinal, B.J. (1996) Readability of patient education materials, *Journal of the Neuromusculoskeletal System*, 4(1): 8–11.

Regan, J. (1998) Will current clinical effectiveness initiatives encourage and facilitate practitioners to use evidence-based practice for the benefit of their clients?, *Journal of Clinical Nursing*, 7: 244–250.

Reid, J.C., Klachko, D.M., Kardash, C.A.M., Robinson, R.D., Scholes, R. and Howard, D. (1995) Why people don't learn from diabetes literature: influence of text and reader characteristics, *Patient Education and Counseling*, 25: 31–38.

Reynolds, M. (1978) No news is bad news: patients' views about communication in hospital, *British Medical Journal*, 1: 1673–1676.

Rippey, R., Bill, D., Abeles, M., *et al.* (1987) Computer-based patient education for older persons with osteoarthritis, *Arthritis Rheum*, 30: 932–935.

Roach, J.A., Tremblay, L.M. and Bowers, D.L. (1995) A preoperative assessment and education programme: implementation and outcomes, *Patient Education and Counseling*, 25: 83–88.

Rocella, E.J. and Lenfant, C. (1992) Considerations regarding the cost and effectiveness of public and patient education programmes, *Journal of Human Hypertension*, 6: 463–467.

Rodwell, C.M. (1996) An analysis of the concept of empowerment. *Journal of Advanced Nursing*, 23: 305–313.

Rogers, C.R. (1969) *Freedom to Learn*, Columbus, Ohio: Merrill.

Rosenstock, I.M. (1974) Historical origins of the Health Belief Model, *Health Education Monographs*, 2: 1–8.

Rosenvinge, H.P., Groarke, E.P. and Bradshaw, J.W.S. (1990) Drug compliance amongst psychiatric day hospital attenders, *Age and Ageing*, 19: 191–194.

Roter, D. (1987) An exploration of health education's responsibility for a partnership model of client–provider relations, *Patient Education and Counseling*, 9: 25–31.

Roth, H. (1987) Ten year update on patient compliance research, *Patient Education and Counseling*, 10: 107–116.

Rourke, A.M. (1991) Self-care: chore or challenge, *Journal of Advanced Nursing*, 16: 233–241.

Rovelli, M., Palmeri, D., Vossler, E., Bartus, S., Holl, D. and Schweizer, R. (1989) Noncompliance in organ transplant recipients, *Transplantation Proceedings*, 21: 833–834.

Royal College of Physicians, Working Party Report (1984) Journal of Royal College of Physicians, London, 18: 7–17.

Rozenberg, S., Vandromme, J., Kroll, M., Pastijn, A. and Liebens, F. (1995) Compliance to hormone replacement therapy, *International Journal of Fertility*, 40, Supplement 1: 23–32.

Rutter, D.R., Quine, L. and Chesham, D.J. (1993) *Social Psychological Approaches to Health*, New York: Harvester Wheatsheaf.

Ruzicki, D.A. (1989) Realistically meeting the educational needs of hospitalized acute and short-stay patients, *Nursing Clinics of North America*, 24(3): 629–637.

Sarna, L. and Ganley, B.J. (1995) A survey of lung cancer patient-education materials, *Oncology Nursing Forum*, 22(10): 1545–1550.

Scriven, A. and Tucker, C. (1997) The quality and management of written information presented to women undergoing hysterectomy, *Journal of Clinical Nursing*, 6: 107–113.

Sengupta, S. and Roe, K.M. (1996) Needs assessment for patient education for people with HIV/AIDS, *Health Education Research*, 11(1): 117–124.

Sheffer, A.L. and Taggart, V.S. (1993) The national asthma education program, *Medical Care*, 31(3): MS20-MS28, Supplement.

Shillitoe, R. and Christie, M. (1990) Psychological approaches to the management of chronic illness. The example of diabetes mellitus, pages 177–208 in Bennett, P., Weinman, J. and Spurgein, P. (eds) *Current Developments in Health Psychology*, London: Harwood Academic Publishers.

Simons, M.R. (1992) Interventions related to compliance, *Nursing Clinics of North America*, 27(2): 477–494.

Sims, S.E.R. (1991) The nature and relevance of theory for practice, chapter 3 in Gray, G. and Pratt, R. (eds) *Towards a Discipline of Nursing*, Edinburgh: Churchill Livingstone, pp. 51–72.

Sines, D. (1995) *Community Health Care Nursing*, Oxford: Blackwell Science.

Skelton, A.M. (1997) Patient education for the millennium: beyond control and emancipation?, *Patient Education and Counseling*, 31: 151–158.

Skelton, A.M., Murphy, E.A., Murphy, R.J.L. and O'Dowd, T.C. (1995) Patient education for low back pain in general practice, *Patient Education and Counseling*, 25: 329–334.

Skinner, C.S., Siegfried, J.C., Kegler, M.C. and Strecher, V.J. (1993) The potential of computers in patient education, *Patient Education and Counseling*, 22: 27–34.

Slack, W.V. (1977) The patient's right to decide, *Lancet* II (8031) 30 July: 240.

Sleight, P. (1995) Teaching communication skills: part of medical education?, *Journal of Human Hypertension*, 9: 67–69.

Sluijs, E.M. and Knibbe, J.J. (1991) Patient compliance with exercise: different theoretical approaches to short-term and long-term compliance, *Patient Education and Counseling*, 17: 191–204.

Smith, J. (1979a) Is the nursing profession really research-based?, *Journal of Advanced Nursing*, 4: 319–325.

Smith, J.P. (1979b) The challenge of health education for nurses in the 1980's, *Journal of Advanced Nursing*, 4: 531–543.

Smith, L.N. (1994) An analysis and reflections on the quality of nursing research in 1992, *Journal of Advanced Nursing*, 19: 385–393.

Smith, M., Rousseau, N., Lecouturier, J., Gregson, B., Bond, J. and Rodgers, H. (1997) Are older people satisfied with discharge information?, *Nursing Times*, 93(43): 52–53.

Smith, R. (1998) Internet update, *M.D. Computing*, 15(1): 10–27.

Smith, T. (1992) Information for patients. Writing simple English is difficult, even for patients, *British Medical Journal*, 305: 1242.

Smyth, M., McCaughan, E. and Harrisson, S. (1995) Women's perceptions of their experiences with breast cancer: are their needs being addressed?, *European Journal of Cancer Care*, 4: 86–92.

Speedling, E.J. and Rose, D.N. (1985) Building an effective doctor–patient relationship: from patient satisfaction to patient participation, *Social Science and Medicine*, 21(2): 115–120.

Squyres, W.D. (1980) *Patient Education: An Inquiry into the State of the Art*, New York: Springer Publishing Company.

Steele, J.D., Blackwell, B., Gutman, M.C. and Jackson, J.C. (1987) The activated patient: dogma, dream or desideratum?, *Patient Education and Counseling*, 10: 3–23.

Stenner, A.J., Smith, M. and Burdick, D.S. (1983) Toward a theory of construct definition, *Journal of Educational Measurement*, 20(4): 305–316.

Stirewalt, C.F. *et al.* (1982) Effectiveness of an ambulatory care telephone service in reducing drop-in visits and improving satisfaction with care, *Medical Care*, 20: 739–748.

Strauss, A.L. and Glaser, B.G. (1975) *Chronic Illness and the Quality of Life*, Saint Louis: C.V. Mosby Company.

Streubert, H.J. and Carpenter, D.R. (1995) *Qualitative Research in Nursing: Advancing the Humanistic Imperative*, Philadelphia: J.B. Lippincott Company.

Superio-Cabuslay, E., Ward, M.M. and Lorig, K.R. (1996) Patient education interventions in osteoarthritis and rheumatoid arthritis: a meta-analytic comparison with nonsteroidal anti-inflammatory drug treatment, *Arthritis Care and Research*, 9(4): 292–301.

Swindale, J.E. (1989) The nurse's role in giving pre-operative information to reduce anxiety in patients admitted to hospital for elective minor surgery, *Journal of Advanced Nursing*, 14: 899–905.

Syred, M.E.D. (1981) The abdication of the role of health education by hospital nurses, *Journal of Advanced Nursing*, 6: 27–33.

Szasz, T.S. and Hollender, M.H. (1956) A contribution to the philosophy of medicine, *Archives of Internal Medicine*, 97: 585–592.

Taal, E., Rasker, J. and Wiegman, O. (1996) Patient education and self-management in the rheumatic diseases: a self-efficacy approach, *Arthritis Care and Research*, 9(3): 229–238.

Theis, S. and Johnson, J.H. (1995) Strategies for teaching patients: a meta-analysis, *Clinical Nurse Specialist*, 9(2): 100–120.

Thomas, B.S. (1990) *Nursing Research: An Experimental Approach*, St. Louis: CV Mosby Comp.

Thomas, L.H. (1994) A comparison of the verbal interactions of qualified nurses and nursing auxiliaries in primary, team and functional nursing wards, *International Journal of Nursing Studies*, 31(3): 231–244.

Thompson, J. (1984) Compliance, chapter 6 in Fitzpatrick, R., Hinton, J., Newman, S., Scambler, G. and Thompson, J., *The Experience of Illness*, London: Tavistock Publications.

Thompson, S.C., Pitts, J.S. and Schwankovsky, L. (1993) Preferences for involvement in medical decision-making: situational and demographic influences, *Patient Education and Counseling*, 22: 133–140.

Thorne, S.E. (1990) Constructive noncompliance in chronic illness, *Holistic Nursing Practice*, 5(1): 62–69.

Tierney, A.J. (1993) Challenges for nursing research in an era dominated by health service reform and cost containment, *Clinical Nursing Research*, 2(4): 382–395.

Tilley, J.D., Gregor, F.M. and Thiessen, V. (1987) The nurse's role in patient education: incongruent perceptions among nurses and patients, *Journal of Advanced Nursing*, 12: 291–301.

Tooth, L. and McKenna, K. (1995) Cardiac patient teaching: application to patients undergoing coronary angioplasty and their partners, *Patient Education and Counseling*, 25: 1–8.

Tooth, L., McKenna, K., Maas, F. and McEniery, P. (1997) The effects of pre-coronary angioplasty education and counselling on patients and their spouses: a preliminary report, *Patient Education and Counseling*, 32: 185–196.

Trautner, C., Richter, B. and Berger, M. (1993) Cost-effectiveness of a structured treatment and teaching programme on asthma, *European Respiratory Journal*, 6: 1485–1491.

United Kingdom Central Council for Nurses, Midwives and Health Visitors (1992) *The Scope of Professional Conduct*, June, London: UKCC.

Vallerand, W.P., Vallerand, A.H. and Heft, M. (1994) The effects of post-operative preparatory information on the clinical course following third molar extraction, *Journal of Oral Maxillofacial Surgeons*, 52: 1165–1170.

Van Eijk, J.T.M. (1998) How can we bridge the gap between health care providers and patients?, *Patient Education and Counseling*, 33: 59–61.

Vanetzian, E. (1997) Learning readiness for patient teaching in stroke rehabilitation, *Journal of Advanced Nursing*, 26: 589–594.

Vaughan, B. (1992) The nature of nursing knowledge, chapter 1 in Robinson, K. and Vaughan, B. *Knowledge for Nursing Practice*, Oxford: Butterworth-Heinemann.

Visser, A. and Herbert, C. (1994) Beyond the hospital: the role of public information campaigns, general practitioners, pharmacists, laypersons and patient associations in patient education and counseling, *Patient Education and Counseling*, 24: 97–100.

Visser, A.P. (1996) Patient education and counseling rights, duties, critics and credits, *Patient Education and Counseling*, 28: 1–3.

Wainwright, S. and Gould, D. (1997) Non-adherence with medications in organ transplant patients: a literature review, *Journal of Advanced Nursing*, 26: 968–977.

Walford, S. and Alberti, K.G.M.M. (1985) Biochemical self-monitoring: promise, practice and biochemical problems, *Contemporary Issues in Clinical Biochemistry*, 2: 200–213.

Wall, T.L., Sorensen, J.L., Batki, S.L., Delucchi, K.L., London, J.A. and Chesney, M.A. (1995) Adherence to zidovudine (AZT) among HIV-infected methadone patients: a pilot study of supervised therapy and dispensing compared to usual care, *Drug and Alcohol Dependence*, 37(3): 261–269.

Wallace, L.M. (1986) Informed consent to elective surgery: the 'therapeutic' value?, *Social Science and Medicine*, 22(1): 29–33.

Walsh, M. and Ford, P. (1989) *Nursing Rituals, Research and Rational Action*, Oxford: Butterworth-Heinemann.

Walshe, K., Ham, C. and Appleby, J. (1995) Given in evidence, *Health Service Journal*, 29 June: 28–29.

Waterworth, S. and Luker, K.A. (1990) Reluctant collaborators: do patients want to be involved in decisions concerning care?, *Journal of Advanced Nursing*, 15: 971–976.

Webb, C. (1992a) . . . or two steps back?, *Nursing Times*, 88(7): 33–34.

Webb, C. (1992b) The use of the first person in academic writing: objectivity, language and gatekeeping, *Journal of Advanced Nursing*, 17: 747–752.

Webb, C. and Mackenzie, J. (1993) Where are we now? Research-mindedness in the 1990s, *Journal of Clinical Nursing*, 2: 129–133.

Webb, R.A. (1995) Preoperative visiting from the perspective of the theatre nurse, *British Journal of Nursing*, 4(16): 919–925.

Weber, G.J. (1991) Nursing diagnosis: a comparison of nursing textbook approaches, *Nurse Educator*, 16(2): 22–27.

Weinman, J. (1990) Providing written information for patients: psychological considerations, *Journal of the Royal Society of Medicine*, 83: 303–305.

Weisman, A. (1979) *Coping with Cancer*, New York: McGraw-Hill.

Weiss, B.D., Reed, R.L. and Kligman, E.W. (1995) Literacy skills and communication methods of low-income older persons, *Patient Education and Counseling*. 25: 109–119.

Wells, J.A., Ruscavage, D., Parker, B. and McArthur, L. (1994) Literacy of women attending family planning clinics in Virginia and reading levels of brochures on HIV prevention, *Family Planning Perspectives*, 26(3): 113–115.

Wetstone, S.L., Sheehan, T.J., Votaw, R.S., Peterson, M.G. and Rothfield, N. (1985) Evaluation of a computer based education lesson for patients with rheumatoid arthritis, *Journal of Rheumatology*, 12: 907–912.

Whitehead, C.M. (1993) *Audit of Discharge Process*, Royal Liverpool University NHS Trust, Quality Department.

Wicklin, N. and Forster, J. (1994) The effects of a personal versus a factual approach videotape on the level of preoperative anxiety of same day surgery patients, *Patient Education and Counseling*, 23: 107–114.

Wierenga, M.E. and Wuethrich, K.L. (1995) Diabetes program attrition: differences between two cultural groups, *Health Values*, 19(3): 12–21.

Williams, G., Pickup, J. and Keen, H. (1988) Psychological factors and metabolic control: time for re-appraisal, *Diabetic Medicine*, 5: 211–215.

Wilson, F. (1996) Patient education materials nurses use in community health, *Western Journal of Nursing Research*, 18(2): 195–205.

Wilson-Barnett, J. (1978) Patients' emotional response to barium X-rays, *Journal of Advanced Nursing*, 3: 37–46.

Wilson-Barnett, J. (1988) Patient teaching or patient counselling?, *Journal of Advanced Nursing*, 13: 215–222.

Wilson-Barnett, J. (1991) The experiment: is it worthwhile?, *International Journal of Nursing Studies*, 28(1): 77–87.

Wilson-Barnett, J. (1997) Patient teaching: a pain management strategy, chapter 8 in Thomas, V.N. (ed.) *Pain: Its Nature and Management*, London: Bailliere Tindall.

Wilson-Barnett, J. and Osborne, J. (1983) Studies evaluating patient teaching: implications for practice, *International Journal of Nursing Studies*, 20(1): 33–44.

Winslow, E.H. (1976) The role of the nurse in patient education. *Nursing Clinics of North America*, 11: 213–222.

World Health Organisation (1987) Ottawa charter for health promotion, *Health Promotion*, 1(4): iii–v.

Yeager, K.A., Miaskowski, C., Dibble, S.L. and Wallhagen, M. (1995) Differences in pain knowledge and perception of the pain experience between outpatients with cancer and their family caregivers, *Oncology Nursing Forum*, 22(8): 1235–1241.

Ziemer, M.M. (1983) Effects of information on post-surgical coping, *Nursing Research*, 32(5): 282–287.

Zungalo, E. (1997) Community based nursing education: creating student experiences for the new millennium, core paper, Nurse Education Tomorrow Conference, University of Durham, September 1997.

Index

Printed in the United Kingdom
by Lightning Source UK Ltd.
111130UKS00003B/5